Mrs. Mattingly's Miracle

Mrs. Mattingly's Miracle

The Prince, the Widow, and the Cure That Shocked Washington City

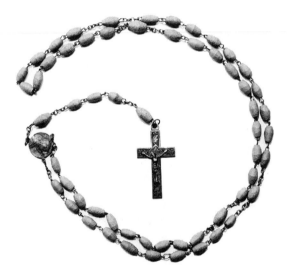

Nancy Lusignan Schultz

Yale
UNIVERSITY PRESS
New Haven & London

Yale University Press books may be purchased in quantity for educational,
business, or promotional use. For information, please e-mail sales.press@yale.edu
(U.S. office) or sales@yaleup.co.uk (U.K. office).

Set in Monotype Bulmer type by Duke & Company, Devon, Pennsylvania.
Printed in the United States of America.

Library of Congress Cataloging-in-Publication Data
Schultz, Nancy Lusignan, 1956–
Mrs. Mattingly's miracle : the prince, the widow, and the cure that shocked
Washington City / Nancy Lusignan Schultz.
p.   cm.
Includes bibliographical references and index.
ISBN 978-0-300-11846-9 (cloth : alk. paper) 1. Mattingly, Ann, 1782?–1855—Health.
2. Hohenlohe-Waldenburg-Schillingsfürst, Alexander Leopold Franz Emmerich,
Fürst, 1794–1849. 3. Breast—Cancer—Patients—Washington (D.C.) 4. Miracles—
Washington (D.C.) 5. Spiritual healing—Washington (D.C.) I. Title.
RZ406.M3S38 2011
362.196′99449009753—dc22
2010039308

A catalogue record for this book is available from the British Library.

This paper meets the requirements of ANSI/NISO Z39.48-1992 (Permanence of Paper).

10   9   8   7   6   5   4   3   2   1

For my husband, Jackson,
and
our sons, Jackson and Jonas

Contents

Acknowledgments

This book has been influenced by significant studies of American Catholicism by such scholars as Ray Allen Billington, Robert Emmett Curran, Jay Dolan, James T. Fisher, Jenny Franchot, R. Marie Griffith, Paula Kane, Christopher Kauffman, Thomas Kselman, Colleen McDannell, John McGreevy, Bruce Mullin, David O'Brien, Robert Orsi, Marie Pagliarini, Thomas Spalding, Ann Taves, Leslie Tentler, and William Warren, who, along with others, have helped shape my approach and provided significant context for this study.

The Cushwa Center at the University of Notre Dame invited me twice to campus for conferences on American Catholicism, providing an infusion of ideas in the early phases of the project. During 2002–2003, I was awarded a fellowship by the Center for the Study of World Religions at Harvard University, and during 2003–2004, another fellowship from the National Endowment for the Humanities, crucial support for which I am most appreciative. Salem State University in Massachusetts has generously assisted the development of this book with two sabbaticals and teaching reductions. I am very grateful for these awards.

Librarians and archivists are essential to the process of writing history and among the finest are Cheryl Adams, reference specialist, Library of Congress; Susan Cirillo, Doreen Hill, Becky LeMon, Martha-Jane Moreland, and Eleanor Reynolds, Salem State University; Lynn Conway, Georgetown University; Robert Ellis, National Archives and Records Administration; Alison Foley and Tricia Pyne, archives of the Archdiocese of Baltimore; Constance FitzGerald, O.C.D. Baltimore, and Miriam John, O.C.D. Portobacco; Michelle Gauthier, Andover-Harvard Theological Library; Mada-anne Gell, V.H.M., Georgetown Visitation Monastery; Ruth Hill Evans and Susan Wolfe, St. Mary's County Historical Society; Robert Johnson-Lally, Archdiocese of Boston Archives; Michael LeClerc, New England Historic Genealogical Society; Gail McCormick, City Museum of Washington, D.C.; Michael McCormick, Maryland State Archives; Jerry

McCoy, Georgetown Public Library; Betty Ann McNeil and Bonnie Weath-
erly, Daughters of Charity Archives, Emmitsburg; and W. John Shepherd,
Catholic University. Thanks also to staff at the American Antiquarian Society. Professional genealogists assisting with this project included Robert
Barnes, Marie Varrelman Melchiori, and Wesley Pippenger. A special thank
you to John Holloway of the Georgetown Visitation Preparatory School
who so beautifully photographed objects belonging to Ann Mattingly in
the monastery archives.

This book has been deeply enriched by the participation of Mattingly
and Carbery descendents and family members: Eleanor Stouffer Albers,
Becky Dittmer, Joe Mickle Fox, John Gottscho, Elsie Harvey, Jake Lay,
Paul H. Mattingly, John Walsh, Suzanne Walsh, and Betty Ward. Thanks
also to Shirley Courtney and Linda Reno. My warmest appreciation goes to
Anne Alexander and Elizabeth Culhane, as well as to Billy and the Culhane
family, who were companions on this journey.

For assistance with German translation, I thank Salem State students
Alexandra Pannhorst and Esther Schleidweiler, as well as Inga Corneliussen,
Robert Spaethling, and especially Emily Westhoven. Elizabeth Blood, Rita
Carter, Elizabeth Coughlin, and Gertje E. Wiersma provided help with
translations of French, Italian, Polish, and Dutch.

Scholars from a range of institutions supported this project, includ-
ing Dorothy Z. Baker, Patricia Bloem, Claire Connolly, Robert Emmett
Curran, Thomas Doherty, James T. Fisher, John Hampsey, Patrick Hayes,
Hans Hekler, Paula Kane, Christopher Kauffman, Kathleen Kennedy, Da-
vid Klooster, John McGreevy, David O'Brien, Robert Orsi, and William
Shea. Thanks also to Bennett Greenspan, Family Tree DNA, and Anna
Marie Murphy, *Boston College Magazine.*

My colleagues at Salem State University in Salem, Massachusetts,
have been both a resource and an inspiration for this project: Patricia
Buchanan, Steven Carter, Susan Case, Annette Chapman-Adisho, Aviva
Chomsky, Bill Coyle, Elaine Cruddas, Lucinda Damon-Bach, Theresa De-
Francis, Richard Elia, Kristin Esterberg, Amy Everitt, Marc Glasser, Perry
Glasser, Carol Glod, Nancy Harrington, Patricia Johnston, Rod Kessler,

Marion Kilson, Diane Lapkin, Patricia Markunas, Christopher Mauriello, Cynthia McGurren, Patricia Maguire Meservey, Kim Mimnaugh, Lisa Mulman, Jude Nixon, Arthur Riss, J. D. Scrimgeour, Earl Sharfenberger, Anita Shea, Jeffrey Theis, Keja Valens, and Pierre Walker.

Friends who offered support include Jill and Reid Atkins, Marita Carroll, Pat Chiappa, Art and Kathy Duffy, Brian and Paula Fallon, Diane Fishman, Lisa and Dana Fraser, Hunter Gordon, Louise Landry, Maura McGrane, Gretchen Mednis, Nancy Pickard, Chuck and Gaye Rawlins, Kerri Rogers, Katie Samuelson, Adam and Mike Stockman, Mark and Jennifer Templeman, Harris and Esther Tibbetts, Peter and Rhoda Trooboff, Norm and Linda Whitten, Laura Herhold and Mitch Wondolowski, and Matthew, Meredith, and Tim Zimmer. A special thank you to Emerson Baker, Elizabeth Kenney, Jan Lindholm, Dane Morrison, and Sydney Pierce, who read the manuscript in progress and offered insightful advice and encouragement. T. S. Eliot called Ezra Pound *il miglior fabbro* (the better craftsman) for his assistance with the poem *The Waste Land.* Frank Devlin gave this manuscript a fine close reading and spent many hours discussing various chapters with me. He is truly the better craftsman. Any flaws that remain after the help of so many should be fully ascribed to me.

During the decade I have worked on this book, new friends have come into my life, but sadly, I have also lost some who were dear. Asenath Blake, Coral Lowe, and especially Christine Rawlins were important in the development of this project, and they are deeply missed. My mother-in-law and father-in-law, Margaret and W. Jackson Schultz, Sr., both passed away during the period I was working on this book, but they were with me in spirit, as was Henry Abram Schultz, as I completed it.

At Yale University Press, I thank Laura Davulis, Jessie Dolch, Ann-Marie Imbornoni, Ash Lago, and Christopher Rogers. Thanks also to Laura Heimert, and special gratitude is owed my superb agent, Lisa Adams, and David Miller of the Garamond Agency.

Finally, a warm thank you to family members Larry, Nancy, and Taylor Lusignan; Penny Schultz and Jody Nishman; Kate, Jordan, Miles, and Ayla Romm; and Carrie, Stevan, and Spencer Trooboff. My parents,

Henry and Carolyn Lusignan, have been a source of powerful support for everything I have undertaken. My husband, W. Jackson Schultz, Jr., and my sons, Jackson and Jonas, are the true miracles of my life. For their unwavering support, I will be eternally grateful, and I dedicate this book to them with love.

Washington City, 1824

The plain fact is, that the progress of civilisation produces invariably
a certain tone and habit of thought which make men recoil from miraculous
narratives with an instinctive and immediate repugnance.

—W. E. H. Lecky, *History of the Rise and Influence of the Spirit of
Rationalism in Europe* (1865)

The mayor of Washington, D.C., Captain Thomas Carbery, left Strother's
Hotel in the heart of the Federal City after a late evening dinner with city
officials and climbed into his waiting carriage. He was comfortably full
on good Maryland beef and oysters, and the whiskey he had enjoyed gave
him a feeling of pleasant warmth against the midnight chill of early March.
He wore a tall hat and handsome overcoat and had an air of dignity appropriate to the office he had held for the past two years, as one of the first
Roman Catholics to be elected mayor of the city. As the party at the hotel
had waned, the conversation of his companions had shifted from the local
politics of 1824 to more mystical subjects. Washington City seemed to be
enthralled with supernatural stories. In particular, the dinner guests had
talked in hushed tones of several recent appearances of a ghost in the Foggy
Bottom area, where the mayor had built a stately brick house for himself
and his three sisters.

    Captain Carbery was a practical man and had selected the location of
his house strategically. He conceded to himself now, in hindsight, that his
choice of a lot was regrettable. When the tributary that used to be called
Goose Creek had been rechristened as the more dignified Tiber River and
walled in with masonry as it snaked its way through the heart of Washington, the capital's engineers had believed that it would effectively drain the
twenty-five hundred acres of the lower city. The mayor himself had invested

in the project and had built his home and his wharf near the Tiber's banks, speculating that commerce from the tributary would be profitably ferried down to the Potomac River. But it was now clear that the Washington City Canal was not an effective drain. The borders of his own backyard dissolved into a swampy marsh. Areas of the lower portions of the city were subject to frequent flooding that left standing pools of stagnant water. Above these pools, residents swore that they saw eerie green lights floating, and tales of the ghost of Foggy Bottom spread through old Washington City.

Strother's Hotel, on the corner of Fourteenth and Pennsylvania Avenue, was located only a mile from the mayor's house at the intersection of Seventeenth and C. But a light rain earlier in the evening had left the road sticky with mud, so travel was slow. Mud oozed through the spokes of his carriage wheels and splattered over the horses' hooves. By the time Captain Carbery reached his driveway, his rig was fouled, and he noticed a peculiar rotted stench that hung in the stagnant air.

When the first shriek shattered the stillness, the mayor jerked the horses to a halt. He glanced anxiously at the windows of his house and saw a light burning in one of the bedrooms. The piercing cry was that of a soul in agony, and though the captain had fought bravely in the War of 1812, the wail sent a prickle of fear down the back of his neck. Another shriek followed, more horrible than the first, but because there was no wind, it was hard to tell from which direction it had come. A third time, the long, drawn-out, painful cry subsided to a moan, and then all was silent.

A stable boy who had emerged from the shadows of the side porch began to tremble. "I told you I heard it screamin' in the swamp, Cap'n Carbery. Haunted, that's what it is. That ghost of Foggy Bottom's been prowlin' around here again."

As Carbery stepped from the carriage and handed his team over to the care of the young slave, the mayor rebuked him with unusual sharpness. He even raised his whip in a threatening way. "Just take care of the horses, boy, and stop chattering nonsense about ghosts. Now wash and rub those horses good. They need to be fed. And boy, see that my carriage is clean and ready for the morning."

Fearing a blow, the slave made a quick bow and led the horses away. The mayor walked along slick cobblestones toward his house. The scent of magnolias filled the air, and he stopped to scrape the soles of his boots on a border of rocks his sisters had placed along a garden bed. The roses, daffodils, and lilacs they had planted had rotted from the frequent floods of swamp water that flowed onto the property. As Mayor Carbery approached his front steps, his sister Catharine met him at the door with a worried brow, and he saw lights coming from the back bedroom where another sister, Ann Carbery Mattingly, lay dying of cancer.

"Was it Ann who cried out?" he wondered. He turned his head to glance back uneasily in the direction of the swamp as the door closed behind him, asking himself whether what he had heard was the unearthly howl of the ghost of Foggy Bottom or the anguished lament of his dying sister.[1]

How the mayor answered that question would partly depend upon his personal view of the supernatural. Did Captain Carbery believe that there had to be a natural explanation for the shriek he had heard? If so, it was reasonable to assume that his sister's terrible suffering during a fatal illness had caused her to cry out and that this sound had been carried outside, perhaps through the sickroom's window, which was slightly ajar. But if, like the young slave who cared for his horses, the mayor was willing to concede that between the natural and the supernatural worlds a window can be unfastened through which mysterious interventions may pass, then he might readily believe that the ghost of Foggy Bottom was roaming the swamp on that early spring night.

To believe, or not to believe? In William Shakespeare's *Hamlet* the disturbed young man famously considers suicide in the soliloquy "to be, or not to be?," but the play as a whole ponders the challenge of credence: to believe, or not to believe? In the tragedy's opening act, the ghost of his murdered father appears to Hamlet and his friend Horatio, both students at the University of Wittenberg. There, Horatio likely would have studied classical philosophy, including logic and natural law. Trained to be a rationalist, Horatio has difficulty believing that the ghost he and Hamlet have just encountered is real. He puzzles over the disconnect between his pragmatic view of the world and what he has seen, exclaiming, "O day and night, but this is wondrous strange!" Willing to make a leap of faith, Hamlet replies:

> And therefore as a stranger give it welcome.
> There are more things in heaven and earth, Horatio,
> Than are dreamt of in your philosophy.

He reprimands his skeptical friend with the suggestion that there just might be a window that connects the natural with the supernatural world, and that we should welcome the chance to peer through the curtains.

Nearly three and a half centuries after the ghost of Hamlet's father exacted a sworn promise from his son to avenge his murder, British writer and lay theologian C. S. Lewis explored the same question of belief in the supernatural that underlies Shakespeare's play. Lewis begins his 1947 study *Miracles* with a story about a friend who claimed to have seen a ghost. Though what she saw appeared to be a ghost, Lewis's friend had long insisted that ghosts don't exist. Her often-voiced opinion was that there is no life after death, what Hamlet termed that "undiscovered country from whose bourn / No traveller returns." Even a ghost standing pale and silent before this unbelieving woman was unable to alter her view. It had to have been, she maintained, simply an "illusion" or "trick of the nerves." Like Shakespeare's Horatio, Lewis's friend refused to believe what she had seen with her own eyes and insisted that the ghost she saw could not have been a ghost at all.

Lewis tells this story to make a point about miracles: experience alone can never prove whether or not they occur. All events, including supernatural ones, must be seen, heard, touched, smelled, tasted, *experienced* through our senses. But how we understand our experiences, Lewis notes, depends on the kind of worldview we bring to them. Whatever we encounter through our senses is sifted through this interpretative sieve. Do we see the world as Horatio does, or as Hamlet? Supernatural occurrences, to believers like Captain Carbery's young stable boy, are those that fall outside of the boundaries of ordinary experience. These can be frightening, eerie, uncanny events, like the appearance of a ghost, or they can be blessings that come as an answer to fervent prayers. Like their darker supernatural twin, miracles demonstrate the intervention of a power not constrained by the laws of mind or matter. As such, miracles are the celestial face of the supernatural: divine, blessed, and transcendent. Supernatural events, good and evil, signal that physical forces do not exclusively control the universe. They suggest that there is, above, separate from, and superior to all else, a power that directs and controls all physical causes, acting both inside and outside of them.

Like ghosts, miracles interfere with nature through a supernatural power. If someone we love is dying, we may haggle, rage, beg, or pray that, just this once, the natural course of events will be derailed. The call for reversal of a clearly foreseen end is a plea for a miracle, an acknowledgment that, in this one case, we want nature to break its own familiar rules. Like ghosts, miracles upend the laws of nature, as strangely as if an apple would hurtle upward and attach to the branch, as if October's crimson leaf would shrivel again to a pale green bud, as if autumn's resting tide would never again ebb from the shore. Believers in miracles, such as C. S. Lewis, assume that God almost always operates within the laws of nature but that the deity reserves a discretionary power to intervene at will. Lewis writes that if miracles are "not improbable," then there is evidence to suggest "quite a number . . . have occurred."[2] But if miracles are, in your view, improbable, then you will believe that they have rarely, if ever, occurred. Whatever your response to the miracles described in this book, it will inevitably be filtered through the worldview you bring to the story. At the heart of this historical narrative lies a seemingly supernatural event: the sensational healing in 1824 of Ann Carbery Mattingly on her deathbed by the powers of a German miracle worker.

Introduction

... remember that a miracle is difficult to discuss or prove. So is a murder.

—Gilbert K. Chesterton (*New York Times Magazine,* July 4, 1915)

Each spring in the Capital City, the March sunshine performs a resurrection. Forsythia bushes along Washington's bustling streets turn brilliant yellow, so arresting that even those hurrying to conduct the nation's business slow their steps to admire them. Thousands of pale pink and white cherry trees, a gift to the United States from Japan in the early twentieth century, blossom around the Tidal Basin at the Jefferson Memorial and along the banks of the Potomac. For the Japanese, the beauty of the flowering cherry tree, or *Sakura,* is a potent symbol they equate with the evanescence of human life. From the earliest days, Washingtonians joyfully welcomed the slender green shoots of crocus and hyacinth reeling their petaled crowns in the gardens of the Federal City. The southern breezes of March that blow through the nation's capital carry with them a scent of magnolias and the promise of renewal.

But in March 1824, Ann Carbery Mattingly was oblivious to the heralds of spring, as she languished behind the shuttered windows of her sickroom, where curtains blocked the sunlight. An acrid stench of diarrhea and vomit hung in the air, mixed with cloying odors of camphor and scented candles. The thirty-nine-year-old widow, sister of Mayor Thomas Carbery, lay bedridden with a cancer that had ravaged her for seven years. In a spare room in her brother's house, Mrs. Mattingly hovered near death. She was, said her doctors, "beyond the reach of medicine."[1]

Already, she wore death's mask. She had been so ill during these last weeks that her caretakers had been unable to turn her in bed. The widow had end-stage breast cancer—a cancer that had spread to her internal organs

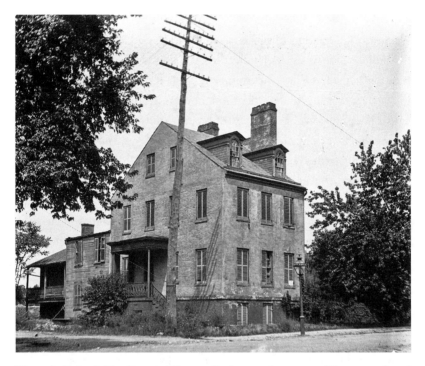

House built in 1818 by Captain Thomas Carbery at the corner of Seventeenth and C Streets in the Foggy Bottom area of Washington, D.C. The house was razed in 1903 and is now the location of Constitution Hall of the Daughters of the American Revolution. Undated photo courtesy of the Library of Congress.

and was consuming her from within. Her rattling breath reeked of the open grave. The tumor on her left breast had grown to such proportions that for some time she had been unable to move her arm and had lain partially paralyzed. Her back and legs were riddled with open sores, which, while she still could, she had insisted on keeping covered up by lying in bed fully dressed. But now, even that had been let go. Mrs. Mattingly, though heavily sedated with a maximum dosage of four hundred grams of laudanum, had moments of clarity when she knew these were to be her last days.

Seven years before, as she was dressing one summer morning in

Thomas Carbery's Washington, D.C., home, where she had lived for about two years, her fingertips brushed against a hardened lump in her breast. A few months earlier, she had noticed some pain that seemed to concentrate near her left side. When she cautiously probed the area, she was startled to discover that the lump under the skin was already the size of a pigeon's egg. Though medical knowledge of breast cancer two centuries ago was fairly primitive, many nineteenth-century women would have been familiar with the illness then popularly known as "the nun's disease," a reference to the higher rates of breast cancer suffered by the celibate inhabitants of convents. Though they did not then understand that childbirth and breast feeding can be deterrents to the development of breast cancer, women in the early American republic had seen their mothers, aunts, sisters, daughters, and friends succumb to this killer and knew that the painless lump they discovered in a breast could be a death sentence.

Ann Mattingly's condition had steadily worsened over the seven years of her illness. The external treatments of hemlock paste and mercury ointment had done nothing to slake the cancer's voracious appetite, and the medicinal mercury she was prescribed may have instead exacerbated her condition. She tried to remain a useful member of her brother's fairly large household, a household that included Ann's two children, her two unmarried sisters, the mayor, and their five slaves. She sewed and knitted when she could, at least until the cancer had spiraled her into debility.

Her mounting physical discomfort during the seven-year illness was accompanied by mounting anxiety over her two young children. Her daughter Susan was nearly eleven and her son John was only eight when Ann had first fallen ill in the summer of 1817. Susan was a kind, gentle girl and a dutiful daughter, but Ann's son had been a source of worry. When Ann left her husband and moved in with her brother in 1815, John, named for his father, had seemed to take the separation quite hard. As he grew, John had become increasingly willful, harder to discipline, and Ann was fearful about his future, especially now that her health was compromised. In her young son she may have seen some of the traits that had driven a wedge between herself and her husband, and she wondered whether John was inclined to follow his father's ways—ways that ran counter to family values and to their Catholic faith.

In March 1824, sensing death's approach, Mrs. Mattingly called her son, now a young man of fifteen, over to her bedside. A brilliant student in classics, Latin, and Greek at the Washington Catholic Seminary, and later at Georgetown College, John had been a reluctant visitor to his mother's sickroom, though he did occasionally help lift her into her chair so she could sit near a window or catch a glimpse of family scenes in the parlor of her brother's busy home. Before she died, Ann wanted to try to find the words that would reach him—words that he might remember later as somehow making an impression, or even as transformative. Though John was study-ing to become a Jesuit priest, Ann had forebodings about his future. She yearned to save him from the abyss into which she feared he would fall—as her husband had—one that involved debt and drink. As John leaned forward to hear her whisper, his face began to fade away into darkness. Everything went black, and Ann was unable to speak. She took his hand and held it tightly but then felt that, too, slip away. Though she heard the door close, she was powerless to call him back to her. She did not know, but could guess, that he donned his coat, left the house, and disappeared into the dark streets of the Capital City.

Later that evening, close to midnight on March 9, 1824, her aunt Sybilla joined a small group at the patient's bedside to inquire how she was doing. Shaking herself out of her stupor, Ann was able to bring her aunt's face into focus and take her hand, pulling her close.

"I am almost gone," she whispered. "If I die, Aunt Carbery, will you love my children and pray for me?" Her aunt nodded gently and tried to soothe the patient's heartache, which she knew emanated much more from the son who had left the sickroom than from sorrow for the daughter who had watched faithfully at her bedside.

By two in the morning, the march of death seemed to quicken. The patient had nearly suffocated on vomit, but her attendants had managed to extract some bloody mucus from her throat so she could breathe. Her two sisters, Ruth and Catharine, and her brother Lewis, had joined their aunt

Carbery in the chamber. Susan Mattingly and a family friend, Anne Maria Fitzgerald, had kept vigil by her sickbed. They were aware that at this hour, a desperate last measure was being taken to save their beloved Ann.

Since the beginning of March, those who loved Ann Mattingly had prayed for a miracle. These were not private supplications offered up individually by her loved ones, but a novena, a scheduled set of prayers that had begun nine days earlier under the direction of a European miracle worker named Prince Alexander Hohenlohe to obtain a cure for Mrs. Mattingly. In the Roman Catholic Church, a novena typically consists of recitation of the rosary, or short prayers offered throughout the day. The nine-day prayer recalls the number of days Jesus' mother Mary and the Apostles spent praying between Ascension Thursday and Pentecost Sunday. On Pentecost Sunday, when the Holy Spirit descended upon the Apostles, they were granted the seven gifts of the Holy Spirit: wisdom, understanding, counsel, knowledge, piety, fear of the Lord, and courage. In Christian belief, the descent of the Holy Spirit on the tenth day led to the foundation of the church.

Novena is the feminine form of the medieval Latin word meaning *nine.* The sacred number nine probably dates back to at least the Roman Empire. The classical historian Livy described the Romans using nine days' solemnity of prayer and sacrifice to ward off supernatural portents, including a mysterious shower of stones, probably a meteor shower, that fell from the sky during the Punic Wars. Some also believe the number nine to represent the nine months of Mary's pregnancy with Jesus. For two and a half millennia, then, novenas have been believed to bring miraculous answers to prayers.

Members of Mrs. Mattingly's parish at St. Patrick's had prayed at sunrise for nine days as a prelude to what they, too, hoped would be a remarkable event. On the tenth of March, the European miracle worker had promised that, if the novena he prescribed was completed, he would offer his morning Mass in Germany for the sick person who had made the appeal. Prince Hohenlohe had already compiled an impressive list of cures, many of prominent European nobility, including the Princess Mathilde von Schwarzenberg and German Prince Ludwig. These days, as word of the cures spread through Europe, the miracle worker was attracting crowds wherever he went.

In the dire circumstance of Mrs. Mattingly's illness, her parish priests, Revs. William Matthews, Anthony Kohlmann, and Stephen Dubuisson, had turned to this wonder worker, a magnetic thirty-year-old German cleric with an impressive royal name: Prince Alexander Leopold Hohenlohe-Waldenburg-Schillingsfürst. In 1822, Rev. John Tessier, a priest from Baltimore, Maryland, had written to Europe to request the prince's prayers for two of his parishioners. More than a year later, Hohenlohe answered the priest's request with a promise that on the tenth of every month, he would dedicate his morning Mass to sick people outside of Europe. By the time a copy of this letter arrived in Washington in February 1824, reports of European cures, and a spate of cures in Ireland during the summer of 1823, had sparked a growing American interest in the devotions of Prince Hohenlohe. The first of the month had already slipped by, so Mrs. Mattingly's priests decided to wait until March to begin the novena and to bring her Communion on the tenth.

Mrs. Mattingly was a member of one of the Federal City's leading Catholic families and a prominent parishioner at St. Patrick's Church. More significantly, perhaps, as regards the miracle of her cure, she was not a cloistered member of a religious community, but a respected Catholic laywoman living in the heart of the nation's capital. As priests and church officials labored to more strongly establish the church in the new American republic, they might well have welcomed the effect that a cure of the mayor's sister could have on the city and, possibly, the nation. Prince Hohenlohe's cures had resulted in a number of conversions to Catholicism in Europe, so it is likely that they desired to replicate this record in the United States. Revs. Dubuisson, Kohlmann, and Matthews, then, dutifully calculated the time difference between Washington and nine o'clock in Bamberg, Germany, to begin their Mass at two hours past midnight in the nation's capital. It was still a few hours before sunrise when Dubuisson hurried through the city's hushed streets to bring Communion to the mayor's home on the corner of C and Seventeenth Streets.

As she watched by the deathbed, Anne Maria Fitzgerald confided to Ann's daughter Susan that she hoped for two Hohenlohe miracles that night. The first, of course, was the cure of Susan's dear mother. The second, Fitzgerald gently suggested, would be equally miraculous: that Susan's brother John would also be cured—of his wandering nature and youthful confusions. Susan squeezed her friend's hand in recognition of her loving concern and fervent wish that both her family members might be healed, one of her physical ailments, and one of his spiritual fragility. John returned very late that night and joined his family and the elderly slave, Hanna, who had been caring for Mrs. Mattingly in the sickroom.

A light knock on the door at about four A.M. announced the arrival of the Reverend Stephen Dubuisson, who had hastened to the mayor's house after the Mass timed to coincide with Prince Hohenlohe's morning service in Bamberg. Inside his coat, he carried a small ciborium, a chalicelike vessel containing the Holy Eucharist that, in Roman Catholic belief, is the body of Christ. Mrs. Mattingly, he saw, was in a "state of extreme weakness and suffering." She had begun to cough so violently that he was apprehensive that she would be unable to take Communion. Mattingly's tumor was so inflamed and painful that she could not move her arm to touch the Host. Her suffering, when the priest placed the Host on her hardened and dry tongue, seemed far greater than at any former time. Later, she would recall that she "calmly and without agitation of mind awaited the final close of my earthly misery." The intensity of the agony she felt caused her to call out and beg God to either let her die or be mercifully restored to health.

"Lord Jesus," she cried, "Thy holy will be done." For five or six minutes, she struggled to let the consecrated bread pass into her throat, but her mouth was so parched that she could not. She appeared to be choking. Then she swallowed.

Silence descended on the room. The small ring of friends at the bedside still knelt and prayed. To Mrs. Mattingly's astonishment, her pain and sickness vanished. She moved her formerly useless arm and propped herself into a sitting position with her elbows, then stretched her arms forward, crying, "Lord Jesus! What have I done to deserve so great a favor?"

The room erupted in half suppressed shrieks and audible sobbing. Hanna, the bondwoman who, at more than ninety years of age, had lived with the family for decades and had been nursing Mrs. Mattingly, whom she called "Nancy," throughout her illness, cried out, "I am afraid of you Miss Nancy! I cannot believe this is you!"

Her brother, Lewis Carbery, burst into tears. Young John Mattingly, according to eyewitnesses, "looked as white as the wall [and declared] no revolution in the nation could have made a deeper impression on his mind." Fifteen-year-old John, born in the second generation after the American Revolution in February 1809, one week after the birthday of Abraham Lincoln, had no direct knowledge of that revolution. But his outburst was strangely prescient of his future personal involvement in the struggle over race and slavery that would bring his own generation to civil war.

Rev. Dubuisson stepped to her bedside and took Mrs. Mattingly's outstretched hand. "Ghostly father," she addressed him in the custom of the day, electrified by the raw emotion in the room and the strange sensation of no pain that she was experiencing for the first time in several years, "what can I do to acknowledge such a blessing?"

"Glory be to God," Dubuisson shouted. "Oh, what a day for us!" Then he asked about her pain.

"I feel no pain," she replied.

"None there?" he asked, pointing to her breast.

"No pain," she said. "Just weakness."

"How did it happen?" inquired the astonished priest.

Only moments ago, she replied, she was certain she was dying. "I offered up a short prayer of the heart to Jesus Christ, and instantly found myself freed from all suffering."

Then Mrs. Mattingly swung her legs along the side of the bed. "I wish to get up."

Stunned, the small circle of witnesses saw her toes touch the floor and the arches of her feet fall upon the wooden boards.

"But can you?" Dubuisson asked.

"I can, if you will give me leave."

Her sisters, remembering how particular she had been about her dress, even in sickness, began immediately to look for her stockings. But the priest gently reminded them that they should first give thanksgiving to God. With Mrs. Mattingly still seated on the bed, they recited a series of prayers, including the Lord's Prayer, Hail Mary, and the Gloria. Mrs. Mattingly's now firm voice accompanied theirs. As the group finished the prayers, Dubuisson consulted his watch. It was exactly 4:22 A.M. Prince Hohenlohe would be just concluding his morning Mass in Germany.

Mrs. Mattingly's sisters brought over her stockings, and her friends surrounded her. She stood up. The small group now regarded her with widened, startled eyes as she walked to the small table that served as an altar where the Eucharist lay. She bent her knee before the makeshift shrine and clasped her hands in an act of adoration and gratitude. Her brother Thomas was hastily summoned to his sister's chamber, where the mayor caught her joyously in his arms.

"See what God has done for me?" Ann Mattingly cried in delight.

Thomas felt her pulse. It was regular and healthful. Her spittle was white, and her mouth, she said, tasted "like loaf sugar," a common staple in nineteenth-century kitchens. The lump on her breast had vanished, and her skin had cleared of the ulcers, without a scar. As her brother later mused on the remarkable transformation, "All this complicate machinery of the human system, so much deranged and out of order, beyond the reach of medicine and medical skill, was, in the twinkling of an eye, restored to the most regular and healthful action."[2] Ann Carbery Mattingly had been miraculously snatched from the jaws of death. From that moment on, she was granted another thirty-one years of life, dying just before her seventy-first birthday.

Because Mrs. Mattingly was a widow of considerable stature in the nation's capital, and a member of Mayor Thomas Carbery's household, the bells of Georgetown College rang out the joyous news. And when word spread that the healing had been the work of a German thaumaturgus, or miracle worker, around whom a cult had arisen in Europe, a slow trickle of visitors to Mrs. Mattingly's residence turned into a flood of believers.

Members of Congress, then in session, expressed lively interest in the event, which took place in the mayor's brick mansion in the heart of Washington, just two hundred yards from James Monroe's White House. Mrs. Mattingly's healing was the talk of Washington City, then a thriving metropolis of more than thirteen thousand. By summer, the transatlantic journals had carried the news overseas. Prince Alexander Leopold Hohenlohe-Waldenburg-Schillingsfürst was credited with yet another amazing cure.

Bamberg, Southern Germany, 1821

One August morning three years earlier, in 1821, the mayor of Bamberg, Franz Ludwig von Hornthal, was awakened from a restless sleep by the voices of a mob shoving through the streets of his city. Peering down from his window at the crowd assembling below, he felt his anger rising. He could see blind people tapping their canes over the cobblestones and the lame being pushed in wheelbarrows and bumped along in wagons. The crowd looked filthy and hungry, but all seemed driven by a force outside of themselves. He knew what brought them here.

"That damned charlatan," he muttered between clenched teeth. "I will put an end to Prince Hohenlohe's spectacles in this city."

Early-nineteenth-century Germany was in the midst of a raging battle between reason and emotion, between science and religion, and between sectarianism and ecumenism, and all facets of the controversies seemed to be distilled in the person of Prince Alexander Hohenlohe. This dynamic healer, credited with numerous cures in Germany, was quickly becoming a cult figure and attracting large crowds wherever he went, like the one gathering at this moment under the mayor's window in Bamberg. The twenty-seven-year-old prince and priest was young, handsome, wildly charismatic, and appealing to both peasants and aristocracy. His personality effectively combined the benign accessibility of a parish priest with the awe-striking cachet of a thousand-year-old name. Once the prince began earning a reputation as a miracle worker, he found himself in the middle of a swirling controversy with his superiors in the church and with his archrival, the mayor of Bamberg, which would lead to his sudden departure from that town during the summer of 1822.

Alexander Hohenlohe had been born August 17, 1794, in Württemberg, the eighteenth and last child of an Austrian general, reigning Crown Prince of Hohenlohe Karl Albrecht and Judith, Baroness of Rewitsky. When Alexander was just two years old, his father died, and his mother subsequently placed him in the tutelage of an ex-Jesuit who instructed him in religion and science. By the age of eleven, the boy had renounced the traditional family career path in the military and had chosen the church. He entered a seminary in Vienna and was ordained four years later. As early as 1815, the young priest was already attracting attention for his experiments with exorcisms and prayer healings. In 1817, he received papal permission to consecrate as many as three thousand rosaries, crucifixes, and other sacred objects. He was described as a man of "fine exterior, gentle manner, a most insinuating voice, and of talents for the pulpit."[3]

In 1821, a devout farmer named Martin Michel miraculously healed the prince's painful throat ailment and strengthened his belief in the efficacy of prayer. Fired with this newfound fervor, he and Michel soon succeeded in curing the seventeen-year-old Princess Mathilde von Schwarzenberg, who had been paralyzed for eight years. This was the first of many such cures, and Hohenlohe acquired a reputation for healing among the aristocratic classes in Europe. Though he specialized in curing princes and princesses, word spread among believers of all classes, and a large cult following arose. Crowds of the sick and infirm mobbed him wherever he went. It was not long before both European church and local authorities were attempting to regulate his actions. Church officials mistrusted the prince's self-aggrandizement, and he was upsetting a delicate balance between secular and religious authorities. But Hohenlohe defied even the Pope's orders to moderate his healing work.

Forced to divert his energies to battle local and church officials, Hohenlohe was soon unable to cope with the influx of supplicants, so he developed a strategy of distance healing. In what could be called the first example of "Mass mailing," in 1821 Hohenlohe began sending out preprinted letters to points around the globe announcing his monthly Masses in Bamberg for the sick. Baltimore priest John Tessier had received one of these form letters, which he forwarded to Mrs. Mattingly's priests in Washington. When this copy arrived in the Federal City during February 1824, Mrs. Mattingly's priests were disappointed to learn that they would have to wait a few more weeks, until the first of March, to begin the novena that would culminate at the precise hour of Hohenlohe's morning Mass in Europe. The widow's condition was deteriorating quickly, and her friends were concerned that she might not survive long enough for this last resort.

They planned carefully, and her attendants followed the prince's instructions to the letter, but there was one factor entirely out of their control: Prince Hohenlohe had abruptly left Bamberg two years before they even began the novena. In May 1822, weary of his battles with authorities, including his nemesis, Mayor von Hornthal, Prince Hohenlohe had asked for a three-month leave from that parish, which he extended until he resigned in January 1823. His new placement in Hungary did not begin until April 14, 1825. Transatlantic communication in the early nineteenth century was slow and unreliable, so the faithful group in Washington had not yet heard of the prince's resignation from his post. So in fact, in 1824, Hohenlohe was traveling and visiting family and friends on an extended holiday. Despite the instant celebrity Ann Mattingly's cure gained for the wonderworking priest on the western side of the Atlantic, given his absence from Bamberg on the day it took place, it is likely that Prince Hohenlohe's famous Washington miracle occurred without his knowledge or participation.

Biographical and Archival Research

The evidence that has survived related to the events in the early morning hours of March 10, 1824, corroborates that something extraordinary took place in Thomas Carbery's Washington City home. Ann Mattingly, whom her doctors had pronounced as beyond the reach of medicine, was instantly returned to robust and long-lasting health. Her restoration is well documented in a collection of affidavits sworn before a judge, and of her full recovery there is no question. Furthermore, seven years after her first healing, Mrs. Mattingly had an accident that seriously injured her foot. In 1831, she became gravely ill with an infection from the injury that was threatening to poison her system. Mrs. Mattingly experienced a second miraculous cure by appealing directly to the Virgin Mary, and her foot healed overnight.

The origin of these miracles is shrouded in mystery and open to interpretation through the lenses of history, biography, and faith. In early-nineteenth-century Germany, Prince Alexander Hohenlohe's reputation as a miracle worker crossed the English Channel, the Irish Sea, and finally the Atlantic Ocean. The prince, then an international celebrity, and Mrs. Mattingly, and these miracles have been nearly forgotten today. But resurrecting these extraordinary events can offer us profound insight into aspects of the bedrock of American culture formed during the early national period.

Who was Prince Alexander Hohenlohe, to whom so many astonishing miracles were attributed? And who was "Miracle Ann," as she became known, a woman who was singled out as the vessel of divine grace, not once, but twice, in her lifetime? Uncovering their life stories offers clues to the mysterious events of 1824 and 1831, and so this book embarks on a biographical voyage to discover the charismatic Prince Hohenlohe and the enigmatic Ann Mattingly. Both subjects of this book, the prince and the widow, present different kinds of challenge in the act of resurrection that is biography.

Because of his fame as a European healer, and his significance as a scion of a noble family, Prince Alexander Hohenlohe left behind many kinds of artifacts. The family castle still stands in the Hohenlohe district, in Neuenstein, a picturesque town in Baden-Württemberg, in southern Germany. Several portraits of the prince were produced and widely disseminated during his lifetime. Many primary documents, in English and several European languages, including German, French, Dutch, Hungarian, Italian, and Latin, are available as accounts of the strange and mysterious events that swirled around him. These are, of course, shaped by the perceptions of those who recorded the supernatural happenings. Biography recovers a life by translating scattered meanings, images, and obsessions into a narrative.

Most people imagine the random occurrences of their lives as something of a coherent narrative, and living an examined life is, for them, a process of forging an internalized autobiography. Biographers, then, work at a remove from the life as it was lived, a process not unlike examining accounts of a miracle in lieu of seeing one unfold.

By all available evidence, it seems that the thaumaturgus Hohenlohe never crossed the Atlantic to go to America, and Ann Mattingly never traveled to Europe to meet the man who forever changed her life. A letter, carried by schooners across the sea, forged their alliance. The prince's instructions in the letter were translated into a ritual conducted by Ann Mattingly's friends. This commingling of the instructions and compliances, though, produced an offspring, the cure, from progenitors whose lives never touched again.

Unlike the prince, Mrs. Mattingly left very few artifacts. She was an ordinary woman who experienced an extraordinary event. Until she was nearly forty years old, no one guessed that anything that happened to her would be of interest or moment beyond her immediate family and friends. The insubstantial details of the first forty years of her life have survived mainly on account of the political success of her brother, Thomas Carbery, who was elected mayor of the City of Washington in 1822. Her husband, John Mattingly, from whom she was estranged, was by her society's standards a rogue. In the case of John Mattingly, subsequent generations may have had a vested interest in disassociating themselves from the connection, and little information about him remains.

Although a large number of images of Prince Hohenlohe are available, I have not yet uncovered one of Mrs. Mattingly. Kate Gideon Colt, the granddaughter of a woman who knew the Carberys personally, left us a tantalizing description. Her grandmother was seven years old at the time of the cure and recalled the excitement and discussion caused by it. But according to Colt, her grandmother's most vivid memory was of Mrs. Mattingly "in the years immediately following her recovery, passing on her way to St. Patrick's Church, tall and slender, with a fine carriage. Mrs. Mattingly dressed in dark colors; her usual wrap was a shawl worn with elegance, and a large bonnet of the poke or 'Calash' type. 'And' said my grandmother, 'I can see her now in my mind's eye, but eighty-years is a long time to remember the color of her hair and eyes seen only under a bonnet, for I do not think I ever saw Mrs. Mattingly without one.'"[4]

In the second half of her life, Ann Mattingly lived in the shadow of her miraculous cure, which loomed over her and altered the course of her family; her place of residence, Washington City; the Roman Catholic Church in the United States; and, I contend, national attitudes toward Catholicism. What is so distinctive about the pamphlets, broadsides, books, and newspaper accounts that survive is that they are anchored in the cure, not in the person of Ann Mattingly. After her healing, Mrs. Mattingly lived another thirty-one years, but instead of enjoying what under ordinary circumstances would be a second chance at life, she was in thrall to the cure, living on as "Miracle Ann," a persona that conflicted with her own wishes and desires.

Supernatural events do not always bring people together. The outcome of the miracle was a church torn by dissent as the battles over the miracle crystallized into quarrels over property and the Catholic position on slavery. The story of the second half of Mrs. Mattingly's life must be read between the lines of the narrative of the cure, an event that lived large in the imaginations of Washingtonians and other citizens. The tools of history and biography can shed light on the mysterious events of 1824 and answer many questions regarding the reception and effect of the Mattingly miracle on American culture in the early American republic. Biography can paint a fuller picture of the two extraordinary characters, Prince Hohenlohe and Ann Mattingly, who are at the center of this story, and help us examine the series of events that sprang from their interaction.

"Some Domestic Cause of Grief": A Note about Historiography

Like most works of history, this one is based on primary and secondary research. The details of Mrs. Mattingly's life are gleaned from materials in private and archival collections, including Georgetown University, the National Archives, the Archives of the Archdiocese of Baltimore, and the Georgetown Visitation Monastery. The information on Prince Hohenlohe comes largely from European archives, sent via interlibrary loan to local libraries. All the details in the discussion of the Mattingly and Carbery families are drawn from archival materials, either directly or with inferences formed based upon historical evidence, a typical practice for historians. They are the basis of this narrative reconstruction.

Inferences are typically drawn from historical evidence, but sometimes, an absence of evidence can be equally significant. Historians are trained to look at extant materials and evaluate, interpret, and draw inferences. However, two significant people discussed in this book, Ann's husband John Mattingly and her son John Baptist Carbery Mattingly, are most conspicuous by their absence in important sources. Though scholars have recently begun to recapture antebellum women's voices through an examination of journals and diaries, it is still the case that information about the lives of these women must also be gleaned from material about their husbands. In this regard, Ann Mattingly's case proved particularly challenging. What struck me as I reviewed hundreds of archival documents about the miracle, whether it was affidavits, newspaper accounts, or letters, is that Ann's husband, who died only sixteenth months before her cure, is almost never mentioned. Nothing is said about him other than the fact that he left Ann a "widow." It is as if he had ceased to exist long before this dramatic event.

As a historian, I began to wonder why. Why is Ann, in contrast to usual practice, never discussed as wife of the "late soldier," "late businessman," or "late merchant" John? Why is it never mentioned that the family had recently emerged from mourning? Why is the death of Ann's uncle, Henry Carbery, who died the same year as John in 1822, more frequently mentioned in archival material than the death of her husband? Why is Ann almost always described as the sister of Mayor Thomas Carbery? It is this *scarcity* of mention that led me to the conclusions that I have formed: that indeed, John Mattingly was not someone of whom the family was proud and that he was already dead to them before he died.

Ann's son, John Baptist Carbery Mattingly, is also notable for his absences from key documents, such as the affidavits about the miracle and his deliberate omission years later from various Carbery wills. A scribbled note in a draft in the hand of the Jesuit priest Stephen Dubuisson described Ann as "uncommonly resigned to her fate—and some domestic cause of grief." Whatever the source of her unhappiness, the precise "domestic cause of grief" remains as lost as the historical records of a ne'er-do-well husband and son.[5]

Epigraphs and Adumbrations

In addition to the dramatic narratives based on archival evidence about Prince Alexander Hohenlohe, Mrs. Ann Mattingly, and the miracle that form the main part of this book are short quotations and supernatural stories that begin each chapter. The epigraphs offer various views and perspectives about miracles, by both believers and skeptics, and reflect key themes that are developed within each chapter. The question of belief was especially compelling for citizens of early Washington in light of the wondrous events that occurred in 1824. The rationalist legacy of Horatio's Wittenberg studies in contrast to Hamlet's belief in ghosts is a debate that was replicated in the Federal City. Enlightened rationalism informed the shaping of the new American republic, and religious fervor fed the varied responses to the Mattingly miracle.

I am calling the dramatic scenes that begin each chapter *adumbrations* because this word, which means to "prefigure indistinctly" or "foreshadow," seems a good choice to describe their role. These dramatic vignettes are supernatural stories that connect thematically or through their content to material that follows in the historical chapter. Though all are based on historical material, I have allowed myself imaginative free play in writing them, so they are much more loosely based in historical evidence than the material on the cures, in which I tried to be as faithful to my sources as possible. The adumbrations continue the conversation of C. S. Lewis about whether or not it is possible to believe in ghosts or miracles. I hope that the epigraphs and adumbrations enrich the reading experience about a true story that is, in fact, stranger than fiction.

Readers of this book might naturally wonder what the author believes about these seemingly supernatural occurrences in early-nineteenth-century Washington, D.C. In *Hamlet*'s opening scene, when the ghost first appears to Horatio and a small band of men, one of them, Marcellus, entreats him, "Thou art a scholar; speak to it, Horatio." Readers of this book might legitimately echo Marcellus's challenge and petition me, "Thou art a scholar; speak to it." Having spent a decade examining the evidence, I believe that something extraordinary did happen in Washington City nearly two centuries ago. In the case of her first cure in 1824, Mrs. Mattingly, an invalid for seven years, was suddenly restored to robust health. In 1831, she also recovered from a life-threatening injury. How this happened, though, and whether the explanation is natural or supernatural, pushes deep into the realm of faith. This book does not try to guide you there.

It does, however, explore territory that scholars more comfortably inhabit. It examines accounts written by contemporaries and later historians of the cures and analyzes conflicting views of the event. The evidence that shapes this narrative is gleaned from historical sources, both primary and secondary, but is principally based in extensive archival research. The book also synthesizes the extant documentation of the lives of the participants and strives to breathe life into the principal characters. As a social history, it endeavors to illuminate the historical contexts, both in the United States and abroad, for these events; and it investigates the multiple significances of the miracles as contemporaries and commentators struggled to understand their meaning. The response to these miracles in the early American republic sheds important light on issues such as race, religion, and gender, central to this seminal period in American culture.

Some Historical Context

Ten years before an infamous anti-Catholic riot that destroyed an Ursuline Monastery in Charlestown, Massachusetts, and just three months before Ann Mattingly's cure, on December 2, 1823, President James Monroe delivered a speech to Congress that became known as the Monroe Doctrine. Essentially, the United States was informing the powers of the Old World that the American continents were no longer open to European colonization and that any effort to extend European political influence into the New World would be considered by the United States "as dangerous to our peace and safety." While the Monroe Doctrine was primarily a response to the threat of European intervention into Latin American countries, it did suggest a conscious distancing of the United States from Old World politics and the stirring of a nativist sensibility that would predominate in the country by mid-century. Newspaper reports of the day confirm that congressmen were among the thousands of visitors who thronged to see Ann Mattingly after her cure. Within months of hearing President Monroe deliver his message, members of Congress were expressing avid interest in the Mattingly cure, which took place in the heart of Washington, D.C.

The charismatic European priest Hohenlohe stoked a spectral paranoia on the part of some American Protestants, one that was violently expressed in the burning of the Charlestown Convent in 1834 and in other acts of anti-Catholic violence that followed. Anti-Catholic commentators feared that Hohenlohe, like the Pope, was a foreign religious figure extending his reach across the Atlantic to meddle in American culture. And like Old World Catholic monarchs, he was attempting to exert his influence in the American continents. In this context, the concerns of one of the sharpest critics of the Mattingly miracle, who called himself "Friend of Truth" and who published his views in a forty-one-page pamphlet, are quite significant. His characterization of the prince as "the long-fingered Hohenlohe" played into Protestant fears that European leaders had the potential to meddle in American concerns. Within this political context, some began to perceive the prince himself, to borrow the words of the Monroe Doctrine, as "dangerous to our peace and safety."

In addition to embodying classic anxieties about Catholicism as undemocratic, the Mattingly miracle of 1824 had several other significant features. One of these is certainly the role of the prince, a European priest of noble lineage, whose pedigree underscored the hierarchical nature of Catholicism and focused attention on priestly power. Tension over the role of the Catholic priest in the United States was already in evidence in the early American church as early as the 1790s. While the moderate American bishop John Carroll (1735–1815), for example, regarded the work of priests as pastoral and communal, others such as the Jesuit John Ashton (1742–1815), a Maryland missionary, viewed the role of the priest as a guardian and protector, preserving a hierarchical view of the priesthood as superior to his flock. Conversations about the role of the priest were connected to larger questions about how Catholicism could blend with the ideals of the new American nation.[6]

Another noteworthy feature of Hohenlohe's many healings is that most of the cured were women. In addition to his European cures, and Ann Mattingly's in Washington City, about seventeen other American healings were attributed to the prince during the second and third decades of the nineteenth century. Religious women in Georgetown, in Portobacco, Maryland, and in Carmelite monasteries were reportedly cured, along with a male mathematics professor at St. Mary's Seminary in Baltimore. Critics contended that only a few of the cures in Europe had been authenticated, and those were all of women. And among the women cured in the United States, Ann Mattingly's healing stood out. London's *Orthodox Journal,* in addition to hailing the cure's providential setting in the heart of the nation's capital, alludes to Mrs. Mattingly's special situation as a prominent laywoman, the sister of the mayor of Washington, D.C.: "Hitherto it has been alleged that these miracles have been wrought in corners, and on the person of some nun or individual of no rank in society.—Here, however, the case is different. To confound the incredulous, God has manifested his power in the midst of a shrewd and sensible people, who are not shackled with restrictions, nor harassed with penalties for exercising the right of conscience, and time will shew us the result."[7]

Mrs. Mattingly's social status and residence in the nation's capital gave her case a special resonance, but the fact that she was female correspondingly undermined its power. A writer calling himself Chrysostom alleged that in Ireland, "only three or four females" had authenticated cures. Even contemporary Catholic commentators were aware of the charged significance of gender in these cures. In 1831, Sister Mary Apollonia of the George-town Visitation Monastery, who had herself experienced a cure attributed to Prince Hohenlohe, wrote to her confessor, saying, "we will have to double and treble our prayers, as there is question of obtaining the miraculous cure of *men*." One Catholic writer in the *National Journal* highlighted these gendered tensions when he labeled supporters of the Mattingly miracle as "ignorant and shallow men, petulant & snarling old women." Certainly, these cures are invaluable in understanding the role of gender and spiritual-ism in early nineteenth-century views of illness and healing.[8]

A recent study of divine healing focuses on Protestant culture during a slightly later period than we are considering, from 1860 to 1900, a genera-tion after Ann Mattingly's healings. According to Heather Curtis in *Faith in the Great Physician* (2007), most early-nineteenth-century Protestants believed that miracles were a rarity and that few had occurred since the wonderworking of Jesus. By the 1850s, however, reports of miraculous cures in Protestant communities in Europe began to filter through American evangelical Protestant communities and sparked a growing interest in the efficacy of prayer, culminating in the flowering of the "faith cure" in the 1870s and 1880s "as a transatlantic and interdenominational phenomenon."[9]

In discussing the antebellum era, Curtis writes, "For women who came of age in the antebellum era, a devotional ethic that promoted passive resignation as the appropriate Christian response to pain resonated with prevailing gender norms that associated true womanhood with self-sacrifice and submission." While, as Curtis notes, this notion of what Barbara Welter called "true womanhood" is well-documented in Protestant culture, Ann Mattingly's two cures in 1824 and 1831 may suggest a previously unexplored radicalism in early American Catholicism, fifty years before the flowering of interest in the Protestant faith cure.[10]

If, as Curtis argues, Protestant "advocates of faith cure . . . contested in-herited ideas about the role of sanctified suffering in the Christian life," what are we to make of Ann Mattingly's double recovery in the early decades of the nineteenth century? Mrs. Mattingly's suffering coincides more closely with the monastic ideal of withdrawal from the world into a cloister. In Catholic tradition dating at least as far back as the fourteenth century, corporeal illness became identified with mysticism. Margaret Ebner (1291–1351), a Dominican nun from Bavaria, the home of Prince Hohenlohe, suggested that invalidism that led to mysticism could be interpreted as a sign of God's favor. According to Caroline Walker Bynum, "patient suffering of disease or injury was a major way of gaining sanctity for females but not for males."[11]

In short, female sanctity became linked with passive forbearance of physical suffering. Ann Mattingly assumed this role for many years. During her seven-year battle with cancer, she was upheld as saintly and resigned to offering up her suffering. After her first cure, she was remade into an icon representing the power of the new American Catholicism and especially the recipient of God's favor mediated through the priesthood in the person of Prince Alexander Hohenlohe. After her second, self-induced cure, Mrs. Mattingly became in some ways a foremother of a transformation from male hierarchical priestly healing to the more feminized healing associated with miraculous medals and the Blessed Virgin Mary, which attracted a significant Catholic following in mid-nineteenth-century America. Both Mattingly cures were examples of unexplained Catholic healings two generations before the heyday of spiritual healing in Protestant America.[12]

Biblical commentators who wrote about miracles saw them as God's messages. How, then, did witnesses and commentators of the new republic read the signs, wonders, and supernatural events unfolding in the nation's capital during March 1824 and again in 1831? It depends on who was doing the reading. For some Protestants, at some level, the events were a threat to the mainstream Protestant American culture. Did some Catholics really have direct access to God, who would act on their behalf? What was one to make of the charismatic German prince capable of reaching over an ocean to touch the near neighbor of President Monroe, who had promulgated the Monroe Doctrine of noninterference only a few months before? The miraculous intervention represented a potential infusion of European Catholicism as the population of immigrant Catholics in the United States began to grow.

For Catholics, the possible readings of these miracles were equally complex. Some welcomed the tradition of the miraculous as a thread to be strongly woven into the new American Catholic tapestry. The links to the European tradition, and the hierarchical centering of power in the authority figure of the priest, were seen by some Catholics as ways to preserve the church's heritage and to promote the church in the new nation. For others, however, the introduction of the miraculous into a nation heavily shaped by rationalism and a Protestant intellectual tradition threatened the delicate balance of acculturation they were attempting to achieve. Like biblical miracles, the Mattingly miracles were viewed as messages to the new American nation. Their decoding, however, was ambiguous and forged by the interests of those who sought to explain them.

Ann Mattingly lived her life during a crucial moment in the United States, from roughly the close of the American Revolution to the brink of the Civil War. During the seven decades of her lifetime, she saw the erosion of religious tolerance and a nation splintered by slavery and race. Her story is one of paradox: miracles that bring not the expected happiness, but heartbreak; second chances unfolding into straitened circumstances; and the public calling conflicting with private desires. Ultimately, the story of this miracle is more tragic than joyous, as it involves lives played out in an era of fading religious tolerance, a family's struggle with questions of faith precipitated by devastating illnesses, and a nation hurtling toward dissolution. The Mattingly family's saga of miracles and star-crossed love is a microcosm of painful national rifts, rifts that could not be whisked away with a miracle but that were preludes to long and bloody battles. The story of the Mattingly miracle of 1824, and its effect on the subsequent generations of the family, is an epic tale spanning two centuries and extending into our own time.

The Prince and the Princess

To know that any revelation is from God, it is necessary to know that
the messenger that delivers it is sent from God, and that cannot be
known but by some credential given him by God himself.

—John Locke, *A Discourse of Miracles* (1701)

Bohemia, 1810

Princess Paulina von Schwarzenberg glided noiselessly into her six-year-old
daughter Mathilde's bedroom at the sumptuous castle of Český Krumlov,
in Bohemia, now the Czech Republic, and stood silently at the foot of the
child's bed. Through the closed glass doors that led to the balcony, the
moon lay low in the sky in the early morning hours of July 1, 1810. It shim-
mered over the rooftops of the Renaissance and Baroque burgher's architec-
ture in this charming riverfront town nestled alongside the Austrian border.
At night, the Český Krumlov castle could be a lonely and scary place for a
child, especially a sickly one whose noble parents took her hardier brothers
and sisters on trips to glittering centers of European aristocratic life, Prague,
Vienna, and Paris. At such times, Mathilde, mostly confined to her bed, was
left to the care of nurses. Her seven siblings grew up with the twin privileges
of noble lineage and good health. But Princess Mathilde was sickly. When
her baby teeth had come in, she had been wracked with fever and swollen
glands. By age two, she lost her ability to walk. While her healthy brothers
and sisters frolicked in the magnificent castle gardens, palace physicians
had tried a variety of remedies, such as salt and herbal baths, to restore
Mathilde. The finest physicians in Bohemia would leave the nursery grim-
faced, shaking their heads in negative response to her parents' hopeful
glances. The child developed a tumor on the groin that became an open
abscess, and she was often confined to her bed. At one point, her mother

traveled with her to Paris to consult a famous physician, Dr. Dubois, who prescribed a series of baths over the years at spas in Cotret, Nice, and Pisa.[1]

Because she was an invalid, Mathilde lived a highly constrained life within the luxurious expanse of Český Krumlov, one of the largest chateaux complexes in Europe. There, forty buildings centered around five court-yards, and its main castle and six-story tower brooded on a mountain of rock overlooking the River Vltava. The seat of the Schwarzenbergs featured acres of manicured gardens with cascading fountains flanked by marble statues of water deities and fish, a lavish castle separate from the family residence that housed a museum filled with paintings and sculpture, and a theater complete with scenery, costumes, props, and machines for special effects.

So when her mother appeared at her bedside in a sumptuous ball gown, wearing a gold necklace and a glittering crown, Mathilde must have thought she was seeing an illusion worthy of the famous baroque theater on the castle grounds. Paulina, a radiant beauty and talented artist, stood before her daughter in the darkened nursery. Moonlight through the win-dow illuminated Paulina's pale face, translucent under her glossy dark curls piled behind the decorative crown that encircled her lovely head. Born in Belgium as the Baroness von Aremberg in 1774, Paulina's elegant blue silk gown set off her dark eyes to great advantage. Its plunging neckline framed a delicately molded bust of satiny white skin, upon which lay an exquisitely crafted gold necklace engraved with the names of her children.

Renowned as much for her intelligence and artistic talent in paint-ing as for her beauty, thirty-six-year-old Paulina was arrayed tonight for a lavish ball celebrating the wedding of Napoleon Bonaparte, the famous French military and political leader, to Marie Louise, princess of Austria. The marriage had been officiated during the spring of 1810, following Na-poleon's string of victories across Europe. Her brother-in-law, the Austrian ambassador, had helped to negotiate the emperor's second marriage after Napoleon's divorce from Josephine, who had been unable to produce an heir. Up to fifteen hundred guests would attend tonight's celebration in the ambassador's mansion.[2]

Mathilde stirred restlessly in her bed, her drowsiness now dispelled by her mother's fixed gaze. She had been sleeping feverishly all night and was under the constant care of her nurse. But in the hours past midnight, the exhausted nurse had fallen asleep in an adjoining room, and Mathilde had awakened to see her mother standing before her at the end of her bed, looking at her with sadness.

"Mama!" she cried. "I was dreaming about the ball! The people were dancing. They were so happy. But Mama! They started to run. They were crying and screaming. And now you've come back from Paris! Is Papa with you? Mama, why were the people screaming?"

Mathilde rubbed her eyes to bring her mother's face more clearly into focus. She feebly propped herself on her elbow and vainly searched the dim recesses of her room, looking for her mother. "Mama!" she called. "Mama!

Hearing her cries, the old nurse stumbled into the room. "Mathilde! What is it, child?"

"Nurse, Mama was here! She was standing at the foot of my bed, looking very sad. But now she's gone."

"Mathilde, my dear, you must have been dreaming. You know your mama is in Paris, with your papa, and your sisters. They won't be back for a few weeks."

"Nurse, I tell you she was here. She was here!" And Mathilde began to weep.

At that moment, a scene of terrible devastation was unfolding at the Austrian Embassy in Paris, where the magnificent ball had been given in honor of the royal couple, Emperor Napoleon and his new empress, Marie Louise. Mathilde's uncle, the Austrian ambassador, lived at a mansion that had been formerly owned by the widow of the Duke of Orléans in Paris's rue de la Chaussée d'Antin. Since the house was too small for the lavish entertainment that was planned, an addition with a ballroom had been hastily constructed, reached by a wooden bridge from the main residence. Painted and decorated paper covered the ceilings. The floorboards were laid on a frame to raise them to the same level as the floors of the mansion. In the center of the ballroom, a large chandelier had been hung, and candelabra

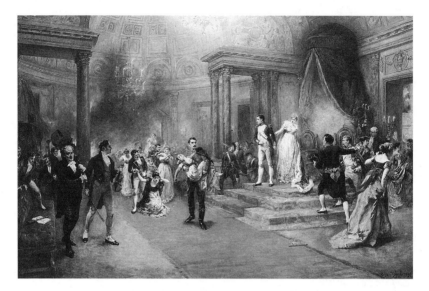

"The Disaster at the Ball Given by the Austrian Embassy in Paris, 1810," by Robert Alexander Hillingford. Image thanks to the Art Renewal Center, http://www.artrenewal.org.

were installed on the wooden walls. A high platform in the hall was reserved for the imperial family. Mathilde's parents, Joseph and Paulina, accompanied by their two daughters, were on hand to help with the ceremonies.[3]

Napoleon and his bride alighted from their carriage about ten o'clock and were greeted by the ambassador. A fanfare of trumpets announced the arrival of the emperor and empress, who passed through lush gardens where mythological scenes had been installed for the entertainment of the guests. In a replica of the Temple of Apollo, singers dressed as Muses serenaded the sovereigns. As they strolled through the garden, music swelled from hidden subterranean grottos. Napoleon and his bride paused under a vine-covered arbor and listened to songs sung in French and German. More mythological scenes followed, including the Temple of Glory, with actresses dressed as Greek deities. Dancers from the Paris Opera, wearing Austrian costumes, pantomimed scenes from the early life of her imperial highness.

It was midnight, and the ball had been a fabulous success. All the guests, including the emperor and empress, were enchanted with the magical setting. Despite the stifling summer evening heat, the musicians began to play a lively Scotch reel that pulled the guests onto the dance floor. According to Baron Lejeune, an eyewitness, Mathilde's sister, Marie Pauline, was dancing with the empress, the Princess Borghese, and a hundred other noblewomen when a candle in one of the sconces near the door fell and set the curtains on fire. Princess Paulina had just presented another daughter, Eleonore, to the Emperor Napoleon, who had descended from his platform to mingle with the guests. Seeing the flames, the emperor's chamberlain and several officers standing nearby rushed to pull the curtain down, but this only spread the blaze, which shot to the roof in seconds. The varnished ceiling of the hastily constructed hall had been heated all day by the summer sun and had grown hotter from the immense number of candles in the hall. Lejeune described a wall of flames that raced from end to end of the ceiling with the "rapidity of lightning and with a roar like that of thunder. In a moment all present found themselves beneath a vault of fire."[4]

When Napoleon realized that the fire could not be extinguished, he escorted the empress calmly into the garden. A number of other guests, according to Lejeune, followed the example of his composure and began to exit in an orderly manner. There was, he said, "not a single cry of alarm, and many of the dancers were still ignorant of the cause of the great increase in light and heat" in the hall. At first, there seemed to be "plenty of time to escape, and the company went towards the entrance to the garden without any hurry or crowding." However, as the heat intensified, Lejeune recounted, those behind began to shove those in front, and several people tumbled down the steps leading to the garden. Lejeune described the panic that further ensued as fragments of burning ceiling began to drop, scorching the hair and shoulders of the women and setting their ball gowns on fire. The men's clothing also began to ignite, and several of the guests were engulfed in flames. Even the strongest guests, he said, "were flung down and trampled on."[5]

Agonized, terrified cries echoed in the garden outside the hall: mothers calling to their daughters, husbands to their wives. The garden, which Lejeune described as being "light as midday" from the blaze, was filled with "heart-rending shrieks of despair" from men and women seeking their loved ones and horrified guests "flying with burning garments from the fiery furnace, struggling to extinguish the flames consuming them."[6] Officers of the Imperial Guard, fearing an assassination plot, closed around Napoleon with swords drawn. The emperor and Ambassador Schwarzenberg hurried the empress to her carriage and then both returned to the scene to offer assistance. The ambassador's wife had fainted and been carried from the hall to safety, but his brother, Joseph, was panicked. He could not find his wife, Paulina. Knowing her eldest daughter Eleonore had escaped, Paulina had returned to the ballroom to escort her second daughter out of the hall. Just steps from safety, a falling beam separated them, and the staircase collapsed beneath the weight of the surging crowd. Paulina was unable to find her younger daughter in the chaos that ensued. Hearing cries from the burning hall that they imagined were uttered by their daughters, Paulina and her friend, the Princess of Layon, raced back into the inferno to save their children. At that moment, the floor and the roof caved in, and both princesses disappeared into the fire. The Princess de Layon was dragged from the flames alive, but she died within the hour.

Mathilde's sister, Marie Pauline, had been seriously injured in the collapse of the stairway. Of the fate of their mother, the Paris *Moniteur* of July 3, 1810, records: "Prince Joseph de Schwarzenberg spent the night in looking for his wife, whom he could not find at the Embassy or at Madame Metternich's. He was still ignorant of his loss when at daybreak there was found in the ball-room a corpse which Dr. Gall thought he recognized as that of the Princess Pauline de Schwarzenberg. Further doubt was impossible when her jewels with her children's initials, which she wore about her neck, were recognized." According to Lejeune, the Princess Schwarzenberg's body was "so terribly disfigured that it was only recognised by her diamonds and other jewels . . . her diadem had been melted by the heat, and the silver setting had left its mark in a deep groove on her skull." The account in the *Moniteur* concludes with this note: "The act of devotion

which cost her her life shows how much her loss is to be regretted, for death
was certain amid the fury of the flames. Only a mother would have dared to
face the danger." Later, it became known that the tragedy was compounded;
Paulina had been expecting another child.[7]

Several victims died that night from their injuries, while others lingered for days, only to succumb in terrible agony. Mathilde's sister, Marie
Paulina, remained in critical condition for a long period. At first, her mother's death was concealed from her, but she read the unmistakable grief in her
father's face and understood that her mother had been lost. Of their mother,
Paulina, Napoleon Bonaparte remarked: "The fire has tonight devoured a
heroic woman." European newspapers carried stories of the heartbreaking
event, and the poet Felicia Hemans recorded the tragic tale of the princess's
death in her poem "Pauline."[8]

According to legends of the castle of Český Krumlov, Paulina's ghost
appeared in Bohemia on the night of the fire. It took several days for word to
reach six-year-old Mathilde at the castle that her mother had died a horrible
death in a fire that killed nine others in Paris. But the vision of her mother
appearing to her in her bedroom on the night of the fire had already warned
her to expect this news.

Würzburg, 1821

Eleven years later, Mathilde found herself at the center of a controversy that
was the talk of Europe. Her health had not improved since her mother's
death. For eight of the eleven years, she had been paralyzed, most likely by
a tubercular infection of the spine. One of the doctors treating her, Kajetan
von Textor, had made the following diagnosis about a year before her cure,
indicating that the Princess was indeed suffering from a serious condition:

> The Princess was stunted in height and small for a child of age
> fifteen, but very spiritual. She was intelligent and mature for her
> age. The spine was curved toward the right (scoliosis). Hence,
> the ribs on that side were forced outward, while those on the left

appeared to be pulled inward. As a result, the shoulder blade on
the left side was lower, the chest and the left pelvis protruded,
while the right side seemed to be indented. Further, her vertebra
were twisted at such an angle that it appeared the spine faced
toward the right. The spine showed an abnormal curvature of
the last several dorsal vertebra and the first few lumbar vertebra.
In the area of the lower vertebra was a hard bone-growth that
caused the patient frequent pain and discomfort.[9]

Recently, Mathilde had begun undergoing painful experimental treatments with Germany's leading orthopedist, Johann Georg Heine (1771–
1838). Her beloved sister, Marie Pauline, namesake of the mother who gave
her life in an effort to save her from the flames in Paris, had died on June
18, 1821, at age twenty-three of the injuries those flames had inflicted upon
her. Yet just two days after the death of her sister, Mathilde experienced
an extraordinary restoration to a level of health she had never enjoyed in
her short life—a recovery from her paralysis. At age seventeen, the invalid
Mathilde, whom a contemporary described as lovely and graceful, with skin
as white as lilacs, was innocent and pious. Like her mother, she was talented
at drawing and playing music. Despite her poor health, she was interested
in a range of academic subjects, including poetry and experimental physics.
She was especially well read in world history and had hired a tutor to work
with her daily in this subject. Her special interests were ancient Greece,
and she was fond of old castles and ruins and romantic natural landscapes.
No matter how ill she felt, she continued with her work and never missed
her lessons, earning her the admiration of her teachers.[10]

Princess Mathilde had arrived in Würzburg, Germany, in 1819 to con-
valesce at the Orthopedic Institute run by the respected Professor Heine.
She was a guest at the home of Baron von Reinach, who lived just outside
of the city. For eight years, Mathilde had been unable to stand up straight
or walk. The most famous physicians of Austria, France, and Italy had
attempted cures, but to no avail. Now, the teenage princess was only able
to lie in a horizontal position. To assist his patient, Heine had invented a

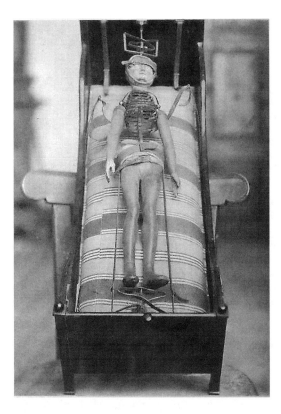

Miniature of
Princess Mathilde
von Schwartzenberg's
orthopedic bed
invented by Johann
Georg Heine, found
in the rubble of
the Julius Hospital
in Würzburg after
a bombing during
World War II in 1945.
Courtesy of Hans
Hekler.

machine that consisted of a small bed that could be gradually tilted from
a horizontal to a vertical position. After twenty months of treatment, the
princess could stand in the machine with her head, body, and feet supported in an upright position. Without the help of the invention, she could
not stand—it was too painful—so she spent five to six hours every day
harnessed to Heine's apparatus. She was unable to walk a single step, and
as soon as she was unstrapped from the device, the pain in her hips made
it impossible for her to stand. A witness later recalled that Heine had been
hopeful that the princess would some day be able to walk with crutches.[11]

On the evening of June 19, 1821, she stood strapped to her machine,
visiting with a friend. During the conversation, her companion mentioned

the possibility that she would soon recover. "O! This will take a great deal more time!" the princess replied. She was carried to the dinner table as usual, and the day ended unremarkably.

The Noble Prince and the Farmer

Prince Alexander Hohenlohe was a slim, well-built man of medium height who favored tailored clerical attire cut of expensive cloth. His eyes were placid when he gave one of his modest smiles, but when his attention was drawn to something, they would fixate with a disconcerting intensity. His pale, scholarly face was an enigma to which women and men reportedly had very different responses. For the most part, women were deeply attracted to his devout and pious persona; men were sometimes put off by their sense that there was something contrived and phony about this noble priest. The prince spoke passionately about his role as a Roman Catholic priest, and he had a reputation for being generous with the poor. His admirers insisted that his behavior was above reproach, but his enemies waited to pounce on any misstep.

Since the simple sixty-one-year-old farmer Martin Michel had healed his throat ailment in 1821, the twenty-seven-year-old prince had developed a close friendship with him. They had first met while Michel had been visiting a mutual friend, Dr. Georg Martin Bergold. Michel had been born August 31, 1759, the son of a civil official, and educated in his native village of Unterwittighausen, Bavaria. After Martin completed his elementary education at the village school, a local priest taught the boy the basics of Latin. When he was about eight or nine years old, he studied catechism with a Jesuit missionary. Even as a boy, Michel was passionately spiritual and an avid reader. His interest in books benefited him after heavy lifting led to a hernia at age twelve that prevented him from doing physical labor. Michel read voraciously in the New Testament and was especially interested in materials about exorcism. The "Gassnersche Writings" of the celebrated exorcist Rev. Johann Joseph Gassner especially fascinated Michel.[12]

Michel also discovered he had the gift of healing. He had learned his techniques from a monk named Ambrosius Fahrmann, who had lived in the region. After forty years of pain from his hernia, the power of Michel's belief released him from his misery. After his self-healing, Michel was able to travel long distances on foot, or on horseback, and lift heavy loads. By the time he met Prince Hohenlohe in 1821, Michel had been curing the sick for twenty years, often without taking any payment. Church authorities, anxious about the potential for social unrest between Catholics and Protestants that might stem from Michel's practice, had ordered him to stop. The vicar general of Bruchsal interrogated Michel about his activities in 1819. The farmer, he thought, had an unusually good command of the Bible for a Catholic and was able to recite numerous passages from memory. Michel told the vicar that the cures were authorized in the Gospel of St. Mark, 16:17–18: "And these signs shall follow them that believe; In my name they shall cast out devils; they shall speak with new tongues. They shall take up serpents; and if they drink any deadly thing, it shall not hurt them; they shall lay hands on the sick, and they shall recover." Michel also quoted passages about healing drawn from other sections of St. Mark and from St. John. When the vicar publicly condemned Michel and charged him with overstepping the bounds of propriety and religion, Michel answered only that he did not cure; he simply prayed for the sick. Surely, no church authority could have a problem with that.[13]

Martin Michel was of medium height, strong and muscular. His thick dark hair had turned snow white, but his eyes sparkled with a youthful gleam under shaggy black eyebrows. His broad tanned face wore a pensive expression, a reflection of both his peasant origins and deep spirituality. The shadow of a profuse beard, which he shaved daily, gave his rounded chin a manly toughness. His attire was that of a simple farmer. Michel had been married for more than thirty years to Elizabeth Seubert, but the couple remained childless. His expertise at farming had made him a very comfortable income. He was a wine grower and had a large collection of bottles, which he occasionally traded with business associates. Once, when his livestock fell ill, Michel remembered the teaching of the Jesuits and prayed for the animals' recovery. They were immediately healed, and Michel had success with curing other farmers' animals as well.[14]

Michel told how these healings increased his faith in God and related a story about his success with healing a horse that had become unmanageable:

> One of my horses had seemingly become rabid. It was so violent that it tore its bridle. Everybody advised me to kill it in order to avoid disaster. But I attempted a spiritual cure. I made the sign of the cross over the foaming, mad animal, sprinkled it with holy water and ordered Satan, in the holy name of Jesus, to leave the horse, if he was the cause of its distress. When I pronounced the name of the Father, the Son, and the Holy Ghost, my horse was calmed and completely healthy. I continued to ride it for many more years in my business.—Later, I tried this Christian method on children and finally on grown-ups. I was lucky, and with the mercy of God, freed many hundreds of people from Satan's snare. After these cures, I felt compelled to help others with the gift God has given me.[15]

By the time Martin Michel met Prince Hohenlohe, he had many healings to his credit. The prince had been scheduled to preach at the parish of Hassfurt on Candlemas day, 1821, but developed a severe sore throat that put delivery of his sermon in question. During a conversation about faith and healing at the home of their mutual friend and Michel's brother-in-law, Dr. Bergold, the farmer told Prince Hohenlohe about his miraculous healings and urged the prince to call upon God now to heal his sore throat. When the prince hesitated, Michel commanded him to kneel. The peasant laid his burly, gnarled hand on the prince's neck and throat and began to massage it. With his powerful touch, the illness instantly vanished, and Prince Hohenlohe was amazed. From that hour, the prince found a renewed faith in prayers of petition, and he and Michel became close friends and associates.[16]

The prince and the farmer had arranged to meet in the small town of Hassfurt to celebrate Pentecost and then traveled together to Würzburg in mid-June 1821, where the farmer had rented a room in the Inn Zum Einhorn, the Unicorn Inn. Prince Hohenlohe was staying in Würzburg with the local pastor in his comfortable and spacious rectory. Beginning on June 14, Prince Hohenlohe offered several Masses in Würzburg while Martin Michel attended to his farming business and traded some wines in the town before returning to Hassfurt on June 16. As was common with European royalty, Hohenlohe was related to the von Schwarzenberg family, and he also knew Baron von Reinach. The prince made a number of social visits upon his arrival in Würzburg and had lunch with von Reinach on both June 18 and 19. Because they were cousins, Hohenlohe was invited to dinner with Princess Mathilde as well but did not mention Martin Michel during these visits. At one of the dinners, a conversation about her grave condition ensued, and after the visit, the prince sent an urgent message by courier to Michel, requesting that he return to Würzburg.

Michel arrived early on the morning of June 20, and the prince asked that he accompany him to see the princess. In his *Memories and Experiences of Priestly Life* (1836), originally published in German and translated into French the same year, the prince recalls the genesis of this dramatic event during his morning Mass: "I found myself moved to tell the Princess that she would have help from Jesus Christ if she could put faith in His divine words, 'Amen I say to you, whatever you shall ask the Father in my name, He will give to you.' On my return to the sacristy, I endeavored to rid myself of the idea as proceeding from an excited imagination. My efforts were useless. The strong impression remained that I ought to go to the Princess and take Martin Michel with me."[17]

It was about 9:30 in the morning. The sky was clear, a breeze blew from the southwest, and the temperatures were springlike. The prince began a service in the little chapel in the house, while Princess Mathilde lay sleeping upstairs in her orthopedic bed. When he informed his host that he wanted to visit his cousin, some servants woke the princess and hurriedly dressed her for her visitor. She drank some hot chocolate, then lay harnessed in her bed and waited, with her governess in attendance, for the prince to come upstairs. After greeting her, Hohenlohe quickly turned the conversation to her poor health and expressed sympathy for her suffering. When she thanked him for his concern, he gazed deeply into her eyes. "My dear cousin, there is a way to help you!" he said. "The help comes from God himself."[18]

He began to tell her of the works of Martin Michel and of his own recovery from sickness. When he concluded his story, he promised, "I'll get him!" and left the room. The princess and her governess, twenty-nine-year-old Nanni Kemper, stared at each other with surprise. Michel had been waiting in the courtyard, as previously agreed, and now, responding to the prince's call, he walked up the stairs. Within moments, the two men entered the bedroom. "Here he is!" announced the prince. Martin Michel bowed to the women in humble greeting and then turned away from the princess and stood still, facing the wall and praying silently.

Gazing at Mathilde, Prince Hohenlohe fervently cried: "God can, God wants, and God will help you. He can, Mathilde, because He is almighty! He wants to, because he is merciful! He will, because He keeps His word. He awakens our belief, hope, and love. Trust in God, Mathilde! You will take off your iron harness! Trust in Jesus! God will help you!" Mathilde, speechless at this outburst, stared at the prince. Pointing to Michel, who still faced the wall, the prince continued: "Princess, this common, but honest man will help you. Not by himself, but through God and Jesus. You will be cured because of your trust in Jesus! So, gain confidence! Have faith, trust, and believe. Get up, Mathilde! In the name of Jesus Christ, arise and walk."

When he finished these words, the prince knelt by the side of Mathilde's bed. Michel turned, and with a cue from the prince, the farmer walked toward the princess. Gazing intensely at her from under his bushy black eyebrows, he exhorted: "Have strong trust! Have unlimited trust! It is not I who helps you. I only have a small part in it! God helps! Jesus helps! Yes, Jesus helps you, because you trust! Innocent heart," he continued. "Unblemished innocence! Clean conscience! Christian trust! You have all this! Now, in the name of Jesus, stand up! Yes, stand up and walk! Get up from your bed! Believe in God! Be confident in Jesus! Love God! And now, I tell you, you are cured!"

The princess, with tears in her eyes, cried, "Yes! Jesus! Jesus!" And with the assistance of her governess, she arose from her bed. Mathilde put her trembling feet on the floor and felt no pain. A flood of strength rushed through her limbs. She demanded that her governess remove the iron harness and asked the men to leave while she changed her dress. When they returned, Mathilde took a step, leaning on the arm of her governess. She continued to walk slowly across the room, with tears of joy running down her cheeks. The princess was deeply moved, and her heart pounded with excitement. After a few moments, she appeared to tire, and her governess helped her back to her bed. The prince and the farmer began to pray again, with even more intensity. Once again, the farmer called out: "In the name of Jesus! Get up and walk!"

The princess rose again from her bed with a previously unknown strength, this time without any help or support. Joyously, she put her feet on the ground, took two quick steps, and then walked four or five times about the room on the arm of Prince Hohenlohe. The governess and the farmer fell to their knees and offered a prayer of thanksgiving, tears streaming down their faces. Soon, the baron's entire household had gathered around Princess Mathilde. As would be the case in Washington, D.C., in 1824, the word *miracle* was upon everyone's lips, and the witnesses were amazed.

Within hours, the whole town of Würzburg was abuzz with the story. Messengers set out for the estates and country mansions of the nobility, and carriages started for Munich, Vienna, and other cities, carrying the remarkable news. Professor Heine had been on his way to visit Mathilde when a breathless citizen stopped him and told him of the morning's events. Heine sprinted to the baron's house and rushed up the stairs. Mathilde was standing before him, freed of the metal contraption he had devised for her, and he was amazed. He, too, dropped to his knees and began to pray. "I will walk to the garden now!" declared the princess, and Prince Hohenlohe offered her his arm. She descended the twenty-four steps of the spiral staircase, followed by the farmer and several others. But when she reached the bottom step, she became fearful, and asked to return to her room. She continued to walk around her bedroom, pacing back and forth until lunchtime. She then sat in the dining room, resting on a sofa.

That afternoon, visitors began to arrive from near and far. They gath-

ered around the princess and stared at her with astonishment. The sight of
the young princess walking around the baron's reception hall profoundly
moved all who witnessed it. Mathilde's cheeks now bloomed with a fresh
rosy color, and her eyes were lit with happiness. Her visitors were moved
with a powerful emotion and humbled by this extraordinary sign of God's
grace. Men and women wept with emotion. On the eve of one of Roman
Catholicism's most important feast days, the Feast of Corpus Christi, the
princess fell asleep in sweet exhaustion. Meanwhile, the entire city was
stirring, awaiting the start of the feast on June 21.

The morning dawned with full summer beauty, and a procession
gathered at the cathedral. Crowds of people, in numbers greater than the
town had ever seen, jostled in the streets. By the afternoon, the streets were
overflowing with pilgrims, and a large procession began at the rectory, to
be led by Prince Hohenlohe himself. His handsome face and dignified nobility drew the admiration of all onlookers. The enthusiasm of the crowd
grew, and some began to shout: "A miracle! A miracle! We have seen a great
miracle that glorifies Jesus and our holiest of all religions!"

The prince's contemporary admirer Christian August Fischer, writing of these events in 1821, declared: "All of nature, it is said, is a never-
ending miracle. We do not recognize it as such, because we are so familiar
with it. Do you know the laws by which a seed grows, or what fixes the stars
in the sky? Have you fathomed lightning at its core? Can you measure the
depths of the sea? Pitiful, limited people, who are hardly certain of your
lives from one moment to the next! You try to determine the limits of the
mercy of One whose knowledge is as unlimited as his power?"[19]

Not everyone, however, was as enthusiastic as Fischer about the presence of a miracle. The crowds soon drew the attention of the civil authorities, who feared that a riot was about to break out. That afternoon, the police
interrogated the farmer and the governess, while the prince and Baron von
Reinach were asked to provide a written statement of the events. The prince
responded in a letter addressed to "Most honored magistrate of the city of
Würzburg," offering this explanation: "The sudden cure of the princess
is a fact and there can be no doubt how it came about. It was the result of a

living belief in the power and godliness of the name of Jesus . . . Whatever you will ask for in the name of Jesus, you will receive!"

Hohenlohe then added this other motivation, in which he cast himself as an intermediary for God's work in the world: "This cure was granted to this innocent for the honor and glory of God. Furthermore, we intended to halt and reverse the decline of faith in our society, one that worships rationality and refuses to live by religion. We can ask this cure of God because he has ordered us to act on his behalf and to save souls. We have been ordered to act on the behalf of our mother, the holy Catholic Church that empowers her followers so much that she becomes God's only true church." The prince characterized himself as an instrument of God's work in the world. Hohenlohe's words affirm his view that he had been divinely commissioned to revive Catholicism in his province and that he understood himself to be God's messenger.

Even Princess Mathilde was asked to provide a written account of her cure. "Nothing and no one has helped me but Jesus and the prayer!" she wrote. Indeed, she was feeling completely well by then, even skipping and jumping with joy. The princess soon felt strong enough to attend services at the parish church of Haug. And each day, as she gained more strength, Prince Hohenlohe gained more fame as the author of her cure. Fischer summed up the effect of Mathilde's cure: "Consider the emotional state of the interesting, sick girl we are talking about. All the pleasures of life that her title and prosperity, youth and beauty, have entitled her to, were beyond her reach. She was connected to the earth only through her pain. She found her only relief in her closeness to God, her only comfort in religion." For those who might not understand the magnitude of Mathilde's cure, Fischer recalled the words of the famous German poet Johann Wolfgang von Goethe:

> Who never ate his bread in sorrow,
> Who never spent the darksome hours
> Weeping and watching for the morrow,
> He knows ye not, ye gloomy Powers.

In Fischer's view, Mathilde's healing brought hope to the suffering souls of the world, which he termed her "partners in sorrow."[20]

Martin Michel remained at the princess's side for eight more days. Mathilde commissioned an artist to paint his portrait so she could keep it near. The farmer then returned home and was reported to be the author of several more miraculous cures. Still, the prince and the farmer had many detractors. Their critics called them hypocrites, quacks, and swindlers. The city of Würzburg went as far as banning them from the city grounds, claiming that Prince Hohenlohe and Martin Michel had attracted "Lumpengesindel, [riffraff], Stromer [tramps] und Bettler [beggers]" to Bavaria and Baden.[21]

Mathilde's orthopedist, Professor Heine, once he recovered from his initial shock at the suddenness of his patient's cure, subsequently published claims that the princess had actually been healed through his efforts, not through those of the Prince Hohenlohe and Martin Michel. But Heine, despite his distinction as the father of orthopedics in Germany, had never actually studied medicine, instead apprenticing as a knife maker. He had hoped that curing the princess would earn him a rich reward from her father, Prince Schwarzenberg, and establish his clinic as a prominent medical facility. He felt cheated of fame by the actions of the prince and the farmer.

Princess Mathilde kept Martin Michel's picture in her home, and on July 25, 1821, she traveled to Unterwittighausen to visit the farmer, which greatly honored him. The princess and her entourage of eight created a sensation among the townspeople of this small village and others who traveled to see the spectacle, reportedly seven thousand onlookers. The princess twirled in dance steps through the room to demonstrate that she had been healed. After eating a simple meal with the farmer and his wife, the nobles distributed royal gifts, among them a silver crucifix that had been blessed by the Pope and silver spoons and china cups and plates. About the same time, the civil magistrates notified Martin Michel that he should discontinue his practices. On August 3, Michel was forbidden to undertake any more cures in Baden. A little more than a week later, the Bavarian government issued an order forbidding Michel to enter its territory.[22]

And yet, for two and half years after the cure of Princess Mathilde,

Martin Michel continued his work as a healer. As late as December 1823, his name was linked with Prince Hohenlohe's in a distance healing in Haarlem, in largely Protestant North Holland in the Netherlands, during which a young girl regained her ability to speak. He pushed himself to visit the sick, even when his own health was failing. In late February 1824, he developed pneumonia and was confined to bed. He was given his last rites and died peacefully at noon during the leap year on February 29. The next day, March 1, 1824, the faithful in Washington City would begin their novena for the cure of Ann Mattingly. Martin Michel was buried in a humble grave that has now been lost without a trace. According to his biographer, Sigmund Lahner, Michel's papers were passed to a nephew, another healer, Jakob Kunz. Kunz bequeathed Michel's spiritual books and materials to yet another healer, Peter Baunach, who died in 1895. In 1936, the same year as Hitler's Germany hosted the summer Olympics in Berlin to showcase Aryan prowess, one of Baunach's daughters piled all of Martin Michel's books and documents together and burned them.[23]

Mathilde's aunt, Princess Eleonore von Schwarzenberg, who was helping to raise her brother's children after the death of their mother, wrote to Prince Hohenlohe on August 6, 1821, expressing the deep gratitude of the family for Mathilde's healing: "Due to your great piety, our family can now enjoy a ray of hope. Through your influence, this child has received the gift of a new life. She will never forget your act of charity, and you will always remain in our prayers." Mathilde also wrote to the prince to thank him and reminded him of his promise to visit her in Vienna.[24]

With the dramatic cure of Princess Mathilde von Schwarzenberg, Prince Alexander Hohenlohe was thrust onto the world stage. On July 21, 1821, Crown Prince Ludwig, later Ludwig I of Bavaria, wrote a dramatic account of his own cure by Hohenlohe to Baron von Seinsheim, with profuse praise for the healer and a request for the letter to be distributed to the public. Having cured Princess Mathilde, Prince Ludwig, and numerous others, Prince Hohenlohe was flooded with requests to come to the aid of the sick, both noble and poor, and word of his wonderworking soon spread across Europe and to the United States.

THREE

From St. Mary's County, Southern Maryland, to the Federal City

A miracle, my friend, is an event which creates faith. That is the purpose
and nature of miracles. They may seem very wonderful to the people
who witness them, and very simple to those who perform them. That does not
matter: if they confirm or create faith they are true miracles.

—The Archbishop, in *Saint Joan,* by George Bernard Shaw (1923)

It seemed that almost everybody in old St. Mary's County, Maryland, had
heard the legend of Moll Dyer. On winter evenings, county residents whispered tales of a strange woman with long, white hair and a flowing white
dress, walking with an enormous white dog through the frozen fields and
woods near a stream named Moll Dyer Run. Travelers on Moll Dyer Road
told stories of how their horses reared up in fright, almost capsizing their
wagons, when a fleeing figure with a terrifying face sprinted across the
road in front of them. Young adults of Ann Carbery Mattingly's generation dared each other to make the trek deep into the woods to touch Moll
Dyer's rock. On its surface was a visible imprint of a woman's hand that
marked the spot where legend says she perished on a cold February night in
1697. Even sober, rational citizens of eighteenth-century St. Mary's County
feared that an encounter with Moll Dyer's century-old ghost was an omen
of catastrophes to come.

Southern Maryland had not escaped the kind of witch hysteria that
had infamously seized Salem, Massachusetts, during 1692–1693. Throughout the Maryland province, a dozen people were accused of witchcraft during the late seventeenth century. Traumatic wars against Native Americans
had caused fear and economic hardship for the colony, just as they had
in New England. The winter of 1697 was especially harsh in St. Mary's

County. Food was scarce, and a mysterious epidemic caused numerous deaths. County residents looked for a cause for their misery, and, it is said, they found it in Moll Dyer. Dyer was believed to have immigrated to St. Mary's County in the late seventeenth century, along with other venerable families, including John and Ann Mattingly's ancestors. She lived a hermit's life outside of what is now Leonardtown in an isolated hut, scraping together a living by growing herbs for healing and gathering forest plants. The eccentric healer was rumored to be of noble birth and to have fled from Europe to escape a shadowy past. She was old and stooped, with a haggard face, and in late-seventeenth-century Maryland, such traits could readily provoke suspicion that she was a witch.

When the epidemic, very likely influenza, worsened and the death toll rose, the town leaders decided to take action against Moll Dyer. On a bitter cold February night, a group of men carrying torches crept through the woods and set her cottage ablaze. Somehow, Dyer escaped and ran into the forest. Panting, she knelt beside a large stone, raised one arm, and laid her other hand upon the frozen rock. There she uttered a fearful curse upon the land, upon her persecutors, and upon all their descendents. Several days later, a young boy searching for cattle in the woods discovered Moll Dyer's frozen body. One arm was still raised in a gesture of damnation, and when they pried her frozen hand from the stone, its image remained there in a permanent impression.

The legend says that county residents brought her body back to town and burned it. From that time on, whenever calamity struck the old-line families of St. Mary's County, they blamed the curse of the witch, Moll Dyer. Just as Nathaniel Hawthorne believed that his ancestor, Judge Hathorne, who had condemned witches to death in Salem Village, had brought a generational curse to his own descendents, so members of the Carberys and Mattinglys who grew up hearing the legend of Moll Dyer were schooled in this lore. Sitting in front of the fire on cold winter evenings, Ann Carbery and her future husband John Mattingly perhaps heard stories of the eccentric European healer who met with an untimely end, and of the generational curse on their southern Maryland families. The doomed marriage, debilitating illnesses, and broken family ties that were a result of the union of these families might have seemed to some like Dyer's ancient curse coming home to roost.[1]

Religious Tensions in Colonial Maryland

About 175 years before the brutal attack on Moll Dyer, adventuring Catholic mariners first scouted the Maryland coast. The Florentine Giovanni da Verrazzano, whose flagship *La Dauphine*, bankrolled by wealthy French and Italian merchants and embarking at the behest of France's King Francis I, was the first European to record an entrance into Chesapeake Bay in 1524. Little is known about the fifty sailors on board, but it can be assumed that Catholic eyes first beheld what would ultimately become Catholic Maryland. It would be another sixty years before English Protestants would welcome the sight of this southern coastline after the long Atlantic passage. On April 27, 1584, two hundred years before Ann Mattingly's birth, two ships left England to establish an English colony at Roanoke Island, North Carolina. The flagship *Tiger* ran aground approaching the coast, and most of the colony's food supplies were lost. After the first attempt was abandoned, the English tried again at Roanoke in 1587. Virginia Dare, the first child born to English-speaking parents in the New World, mysteriously vanished from the island without a trace sometime before her third birthday, along with 110 of her fellow colonists. Other English settlers soon replaced the lost ones and were followed by many more. In 1607, the Englishman John Smith, known for his friendship with Pocahontas, helped found a successful settlement in Virginia and mapped Chesapeake Bay.

More than two decades after the founding of Jamestown, in 1631, an Anglican from Virginia, William Claiborne, opened a fur trading post on Kent Island in Chesapeake Bay, becoming the first European known to settle in Maryland. The following year, George Calvert, First Baron Baltimore and a recent convert to Roman Catholicism, obtained a charter from King Charles I that granted feudal rights to the land north of the Potomac River. Astutely, he named the new colony in honor of the king's Catholic wife, Henrietta Maria. But before colonization of Maryland could begin, the first Lord Baltimore died. He left the grant to his son, Cecilius, Second Baron Baltimore. Since the Maryland charter did not expressly prohibit the establishment of non-Protestant churches, Cecilius Calvert encouraged fellow Catholics, who had been facing increasing persecution in England, to settle there. He hoped to create both a refuge and a profitable venture, so he also encouraged Protestant immigration.

Protestants and Catholics together established Maryland's first town, St. Mary's, in 1634. Arriving in the *Ark* and the *Dove,* they chose a location high on a bluff near the point where the Potomac River flows into Chesapeake Bay, where Verrazzano's *Dauphine* had sailed more than a century before. This new colony flourished. Liberal economic and political incentives promoted the growth of independent farms and the establishment within a year of Maryland's first legislature, the House of Delegates, which convened in 1635. Relatively spared from Indian attack and able to quickly establish reliable food sources, Maryland settlers benefited from trade with Virginia and from the largess of Lord Baltimore, who personally supported the settlers' early financial needs. Ann Carbery Mattingly's ancestor, William Bretton, was among the first settlers, arriving in 1637.

As Baltimore welcomed all Christian sects in his province, the Protestants soon outnumbered the Catholics of Maryland, and a cold current of religious strife began to trouble this new colony. Within eight years of its founding, Catholics were outnumbered three to one. Calvert turned to the Maryland General Assembly, in which William Bretton served, to ensure passage in 1649 of the Toleration Act. This famous document asserts that "no person . . . in this province professing to believe in Jesus Christ shall . . . be in any ways troubled, molested, or discountenanced for . . . his or her religion . . . so that they be not unfaithful to the Lord Proprietary, or molest or conspire against the civil Government established in this Province."[2] Although this act was the first act of religious toleration passed into law in the American colonies, thirteen years earlier, Roger Williams had founded Rhode Island on principles of religious toleration more complete than those of the Maryland act. By mandating belief in the Christian

God, Lord Baltimore's act would have condemned Jews or freethinkers to death.

Elsewhere in the colonies, the Puritans, who had fled England to gain their own religious freedom, continued to persecute those of other faiths. They could not tolerate the Church of England, mainly because they believed it remained too closely tied to its mother church, the Roman Catholic Church. Some Puritans at first remained members of the Anglican Church, hoping to reform it from within, but by the 1640s, others had broken off into newly formed independent churches. This ancient rivalry between the mother church and her children, and among those children, crossed the Atlantic on European ships drawing their currents westward from the continent. By the time Verrazzano had set sail on *La Dauphine,* a revolution was already under way in Europe. Just seven years before the arrival of *La Dauphine* in the New World, Martin Luther had posted his ninety-five theses on the church door in Wittenberg, Germany, sparking the Protestant Reformation. In the German cradle of the Reformation, clashing ideologies of old Catholicism and the new Protestantism became a deep struggle between cultures, and religious intolerance was carried to the New World.

This duel between Christian sects quickly took on a much larger dimension than debates over the intricacies of liturgical belief or ritual. It became a war over the future of the Western world. As European religious historian Manuel Borutta puts it, the "static, historyless Catholic world served as a foil to the construction of a modern identity that was secular but confessionally coloured," that is, Protestant, in its orientation. Borutta goes on to note that in the wake of the Reformation, Protestantism began to be perceived as compatible with modernity and Catholicism as "modernity's other." The hierarchy of the European Catholic Church contributed to this perception by consistently marginalizing promodern forces within its ranks.[3]

Religiously inflected debates over the formation of the modern world that raged in post-Reformation Europe became cultural cargo transported by transatlantic carracks to the eastern seaboard of colonial America. Bronzed sailors handed this invisible cargo out of the holds of their ships along with supplies for the new settlements. With the first spades turning the dirt for corn and wheat, flax and cotton, these ideas were planted deep into the virgin soil. They wove themselves firmly into the first cloth of American culture, a thread so familiar as to be nearly unnoticeable. The colonists of the *Mayflower* and the *Arbella* conceived of their Massachusetts settlements as the establishment of a city upon a hill, an ideal community that would serve as a model for the corrupt English across the Atlantic to imitate. The Maryland Catholics and Protestants of the *Ark* and *Dove* together founded St. Mary's, another city upon a hill.

In order to help ensure peace and prosperity, the *Ark* and the *Dove* carried, in addition to supplies and settlers, several cannons that defended the colony on sea and land. When the royal governor Francis Nicholson removed the capital of the province from St. Mary's to Annapolis in 1694, these cannons, five in number, were left exposed to winds and weather on Fort Point. While the cannons likely stood when Moll Dyer's house was attacked in 1697, the erosion of the riverbank by storms and wind eventually caused them to be submerged in the waters of the St. Mary's River. By the early nineteenth century, they lay in about three or four feet of water, about 150 yards from the shore. There they would remain until 1822, when Ann Carbery Mattingly's brother, Mayor Captain Thomas Carbery, recovered them.[4]

Ann Carbery Mattingly's Early Years, 1784–1803

Ann Carbery Mattingly was born in 1784 in St. Mary's County, Maryland, home to some of the country's oldest Catholic families and accessible to Washington, D.C., by a short boat trip up the Potomac River. Her paternal great-great-grandfather, John Baptist Carbery, born before 1647, was a native of Dublin, Ireland, and arrived in Maryland in 1690, half a century after the colony was founded. Members of the Carbery family lived on the lands surrounding the ancient Carbury Castle near Dublin, where some of them supported the exiled Catholic monarch, James II, who was defeated at the Battle of the Boyne on July 1, 1690. Irishmen who had fought for the Catholic monarch were offered free passage to France. Carbery family biographer Rose Martin notes that John Baptist Carbery's name does not appear on passenger lists of British vessels sailing to America and suggests that he likely sailed from France to the West Indies, where he embarked for Maryland, and married Ann Thompson.[5]

Their son, John Baptist Carbery, was born in 1660 and in 1692 married a young widow, Elizabeth Guibert Scott, daughter of a prosperous local French farmer and widow of Cuthbert Scott. About five years into their marriage, Elizabeth died, before having fully administered the estate of her first husband. John Baptist Carbery, who was the administrator of the estate of Elizabeth, also was granted *de bonis non administratis,* Latin for "of goods not administered." He was thus charged with the responsibility to administer what was as yet unsettled in the estate of Cuthbert Scott. After a contentious court battle with Scott's sister and her husband, a ruling was made in favor of John Baptist Carbery, thus ending the first of many legal battles by generations of Carberys.[6]

By 1712, John Baptist Carbery, Gentleman, owned twenty-one thousand acres of land at upper New Town in St. Mary's County, a property he named Hopton Park. Upon his death, sometime before 1729, his estate passed to his son, twenty-nine-year-old John Baptist Carbery, Ann's grandfather. He was already married to Mary Thompson, a descendent of William Bretton. Bretton's Bay, near New Town, was named in his honor. John Baptist and Mary Thompson Carbery were the parents of twelve children, nine of whom survived into adulthood. One of their middle children, Thomas Carbery, was Ann's father, born about 1745. The bondwoman Hanna, likely born at Hopton Park, would live with the Carbery family for a century.[7]

Thomas Carbery Sr. was a timber merchant and likely traveled to the wildernesses of North Carolina on business, where he met his future wife, Mary Asenath Simmons, born about 1757, making her at least ten years younger than her husband. Onslow County, in coastal North Carolina, fronts thirty miles on the Atlantic Ocean, with a navigable river, now called the Long River, running forty miles into the center of the county. Sailing south from the coast of Maryland to North Carolina, Thomas Carbery would have known that the forests of Onslow County were filled with old-growth longleaf pine trees. These timberlands were a strong draw for an ambitious merchant like Thomas. Longleaf pine is a valuable source of naval stores, such as resin, turpentine, and timber, needed by merchants and the navy for their ships. Boards cut from virgin timber could be as wide as three feet and were highly valued for their multiple potential uses.

While in Onslow County, Thomas Sr. likely met the family of Henry Simmons and his daughters. The North Carolina Early Census Index for Onslow County for 1769–1770 lists Henry Simmons as head of household. According to documents in the Visitation Monastery archive in Washington, D.C., Ann Carbery's oldest sister, Mary Carbery, later Sister Eleonora of the Roman Catholic Carmelite order, was born in North Carolina. Interestingly, these documents state that Mary's mother is Catherine Simmons, daughter of Henry Simmons. This evidence suggests the possibility that Mary's mother Catherine died, possibly in childbirth, and that Thomas then married Catherine's sister or relative Mary Asenath Simmons in North Carolina, without benefit of a priest nearby. The couple traveled back to St. Mary's County, where they raised a large family of nine children on a farm subdivided from the family land at Hopton Park.

Ann was born on March 17, 1784, St. Patrick's Day, an auspicious omen of her future connection with St. Patrick's Church in Washington, D.C. Her birthday coincided with the St. Patrick's Day celebration in New York City, a day marked with fife and drum music and a banquet held in lower Manhattan. In St. Mary's County, Ann's family, including her four brothers and sisters (Mary, age nine; John Baptist, seven; Martha, five; and Ruth, about four), welcomed the new addition to the family. Thomas Sr. and his wife, Mary Asenath, were likely thrilled that the new baby, who was nicknamed Nancy, had been born in early spring and looked forward to the coming of milder weather, since the winter season had been brutally harsh.

Throughout North America, the winter of 1784 had been the longest and coldest on record, following the eight-month cataclysmic eruption of the Laki volcanic fissure in Iceland. The ash and gasses emitted helped produce the longest period of below-zero temperatures on record in New England, the deepest snow accumulation in New Jersey, and the most extensive duration of a freeze-over in the Chesapeake Bay. In Charleston, South Carolina, citizens bundled up to ice skate on the frozen harbor, and ice chunks floated in the Gulf of Mexico. A monster snowstorm buried the South, and the Mississippi River froze at New Orleans. The effects of the Iceland eruption on climate and agriculture are estimated to have killed up to two million people globally, and some say the resulting famines in Europe helped precipitate the French Revolution.

The summer Ann was conceived, a heavy fog from the volcano shrouded North America, alarming farmers, including Ann's family at Hopton Park. Benjamin Franklin analyzed these worrisome climate changes in a lecture he gave in 1784:

> During several of the summer months of the year 1783, when the effect of the sun's rays to heat the earth in these northern regions should have been greater, there existed a constant fog over all Europe, and a great part of North America. This fog was of a permanent nature; it was dry, and the rays of the sun seemed to have little effect towards dissipating it, as they easily do a moist fog, arising from water. They were indeed rendered so faint in passing through it, that when collected in the focus of a burning glass they would scarce kindle brown paper. Of course, their summer effect in heating the Earth was exceedingly diminished. Hence the surface was early frozen. Hence the first snows remained on it unmelted, and received continual additions. Hence the air was more chilled, and the winds more severely cold. Hence perhaps the winter of 1783–4 was more severe than any that had happened for many years.

Ann Mattingly's conception and birth, then, occurred during an intense period of meteorological change. This might help explain why family members thought she was destined for something exceptional, a comment her uncle Henry Carbery was fond of making about his favorite niece.[8]

In addition to the bizarre weather, Roman Catholicism in Maryland had other challenges in 1784–1785. The Reverend John Carroll wrote a report on the condition of the church in America to Cardinal Antonelli, Prefect of the Propaganda in Rome. He warned of the imminent danger of the appointment of a foreign superior, a vicar apostolic, for the emerging American nation, advocating instead for local rule. Carroll reported that in Maryland in 1785, there were "about 15,800 Catholics; of these there are about 9,000 freemen, adults or over twelve years of age; children under that age, about 3,000; and about that number of slaves of all ages of African origin, called negroes." There were only nineteen priests in the state to serve this large population, and Carroll detailed the result: "In Maryland a few of the leading more wealthy families still profess the Catholic faith introduced at the very foundation of the province by their ancestors. The greater part of them are planters. . . . As for piety, they are for the most part sufficiently assiduous in the exercises of religion and in frequenting the sacraments, but they lack that fervor, which frequent appeals to the sentiment of piety usually produce, as many congregations hear the word of God only once a month, and sometimes only once in two months. We are reduced to this by want of priests, by the distance of congregations from each other and by the difficulty of traveling."[9]

Although Carroll found that the Catholics of Maryland maintained the necessary exercises of religion, despite being deprived of enough priests for their numbers, he was concerned that their brand of spirituality lacked "fervor." According to historian Joseph Chinnici, *fervor,* for Carroll, meant "interiority, a piety centered in the will and its dispositions." Carroll bemoaned a lack of warmth and passion in Maryland Catholics and wished to foster there a deeper, heartfelt belief in Jesus Christ. He also was attempting to achieve a difficult balance for his small Catholic flock in eighteenth-century Maryland: a conservative Federalism "committed to the acceptance of religious pluralism but conscious of the need for an aristocracy of virtue and an insistence on the institutions of religion." Carroll's foundational ideas for American Catholicism in the early American republic were drawn from three main streams in post-Reformation spirituality. These were the humanistic traditions of the French, with an emphasis on free will, conscience, and interiority; the English Catholic tradition of the seventeenth and eighteenth centuries, which shied away from miracle-mongering and adulation of the Virgin Mary; and the tradition of St. Ignatius of Loyola (1491–1556), which was centered in a tolerance of religious pluralism. Ann Carbery was born into a Catholic family strongly shaped by these traditions.[10]

Carroll had been concerned that the shortage of priests gave rise to "abuses" that had sprung up in the Catholic population: "unavoidable intercourse with non-Catholics . . . more free intercourse between young people of opposite sexes than is compatible with chastity in mind and body; too great fondness for dances and similar amusements; and an incredible eagerness, especially in girls, for reading love stories which are brought over in great quantities from Europe. Then among other things, a general lack of care in instructing their children and especially the negro slaves in their religion, as these people are kept constantly at work, so that they rarely hear any instructions from the priest . . . and most of them are consequently very dull in faith and depraved in morals." The concern about intermarriage with non-Catholics was so strong that it loosened the taboo against intermarriage with relatives, giving rise to a saying in southern Maryland: "Better to be a little too close in blood than too far apart in religion."[11]

Ann would have enjoyed a pleasant childhood on her family's southern Maryland plantation. Hopton Park had a windmill that powered the plantation's flourmill. Fields of green tobacco and Indian corn stretched out over the flat farmland. The broad and sparkling Potomac River was only a country mile away, with tobacco boats crowding its bustling wharves. Like generations of plantation children before her, Ann would have spent summers picking wild berries and scouring the woods for nuts in the fall. Girls in southern Maryland would be given tasks such as carding, wool winding, quilting, and stitching, skills at which Ann became proficient. She learned to spin and weave, sew and mend, and how to make candles and soap. She assisted in the kitchen, making preserves from the abundant farm produce. She would also need to help visit and care for the six slaves that her family owned by the time Ann turned sixteen.[12]

Once her chores were complete, Ann could roam the woods and play in the streams of the plantation with her sisters, Catharine and Ruth, who were close in age, and with her little brother Thomas, upon whom the sisters doted. As she grew, she would have attended parties at other local manors and gone on hayrides and picnics in the summer. In the winter, there would be sleigh rides and preparation for the great feast days. At Christmas, the traditional meal was a turkey plumped with oysters or chestnuts; for Easter, the large extended families dined on ham stuffed with greens. Her eldest half-sister, Mary, had followed the steps of their aunt Elizabeth, the first professed nun in the United States, into the Carmelites. Ann's friends valued her hospitality and charity and praised her sprightly disposition. Family members were impressed with her "fine penetrating mind—even in her youth." She was a favorite of the priest at St. Xavier's, described as "quite unaffected in her devotion" and most "anxious to comply with the rules of the church."[13]

This glimpse into a facet of Maryland Catholic girlhood, the reading of European novels and charges of careless attention to child rearing, raises interesting questions about the youth of Ann Carbery in the final decade of the eighteenth century. Certainly, Ann was literate and able to write fluidly with good penmanship. Whether or not such European novels were available to her in late-eighteenth-century St. Mary's County is difficult to ascertain. If, indeed, young Ann had her head filled with ideas about romantic love from novels and was permitted free interaction with the young men of her neighborhood, it will likely never be known. Young men and women in turn-of-the-nineteenth-century Maryland attended dances and other social activities with loose supervision from adults. This, combined with ideas about romantic trysts picked up from novels, could be an inducement to plunge headlong into a disastrous marriage.

Ann and her sisters no doubt enjoyed their share of beaux and parties, but her carefree childhood days would end at age nineteen, when she became the wife of John Mattingly. That morning, November 9, 1803, the sun was hidden behind a peculiar red fog that was chased away in the afternoon by a strong northwest wind. Ann and John were married in St. Xavier's Church, a little wooden chapel with a pointed bell tower, where her ancestor had been an important benefactor. William Bretton had donated the land upon which the church was built and had sold his 750-acre plantation to the Jesuits at Newtown in exchange for forty thousand pounds of tobacco. John Mattingly's family was another old-line St. Mary's County family, descended from Thomas Mattingly, who originated in England, and traveled to Maryland on the *Arc* or the *Dove*. Both the Carberys and Mattinglys were living in St. Mary's County when Moll Dyer placed her legendary curse on all the residents and their descendents.[14]

The scarcity of priests for the number of Catholics in Maryland certainly meant that many marriages were consummated without the full sacramental sanction of the Catholic Church, as was the marriage of Ann's own parents, Thomas and Mary Aseneth. In 1791, John Carroll, now a bishop, issued a "Circular on Christian Marriage" that underscored the sacramental nature of Catholic marriage:

> When Christ honored the institution of marriage by raising it
> to the dignity and sanctity of a sacrament, he intended to cre-
> ate in all who were to enter into that state a great respect for
> it, and to lay on them an obligation of preparing themselves
> for it, by purifying their consciences and disposing of them
> worthily to receive abundant communications of divine grace.
> He subjected thereby to the authority and jurisdiction of his
> Church the manner and rites of its celebration, lest any should
> violate and profane so holy an institution by engaging in mar-
> riage without due consideration of its sanctity and obligations.
> . . . [L]ately some of the congregation have been so regardless
> of their duty in this respect, as to recur to the ministry of those
> whom the Catholic Church never honored with the commission
> of administering marriage. The[se] persons . . . hereby rendered
> themselves guilty of a sacrilegious profanation of a most holy
> institution at the very moment of their marriage. It must be left
> to themselves to consider, whether they can expect much happi-
> ness in a state into which they entered by committing an offence
> so grievous and dangerous to their faith.[15]

The circular, then, clearly emphasized the importance of Catholics being married within the Catholic Church and was issued to stem a tide of indiscretions in part created by the shortage of priests. In a time when so many marriages were being made outside the church, Ann Carbery likely took pride in the fact that her marriage to John Mattingly, at least, carefully and dutifully observed Catholic teaching. The sanctity of the sacrament, with its emphasis on respect for marriage and purification of conscience, may have made less of an impression on the groom than on the bride. Though John and Ann's marriage had been properly blessed by a Roman Catholic priest, the couple's happiness together would become compromised.

We do not know the circumstances of Ann Carbery and John Mattingly's courtship, partly because John has remained so elusive. The most reliable evidence suggests that he was the son of James Barton Mattingly and Mildred Nevitt, sister of the Revolutionary War hero Joseph Nevitt, who died in Washington, D.C., in 1833. The 1800 Federal Census of St. Mary's County shows Ann's family, listed as the household of Thomas Carbury [sic], living in close proximity to two Mattingly families, with the heads of household named Thomas and John. The census lists just one female child younger than the age of ten, probably Pann Mattingly, and one slave in the family of John's father, Barton Mattingly. John's family was far less affluent than the Carberys.[16]

After the death of John's mother, Barton had married a widow, Jemima Sticklin Watts, in 1795. The other four children of James Barton Mattingly and Mildred Nevitt, Stephen, Thomas, John, and Ann, are not listed as living with Barton and Jemima in 1800. There are also numerous other Mattingly families living in St. Mary's County in 1800. How Ann and John met is unknown, but we can imagine them, like most couples of their day, chatting at a country dance, enjoying a moonlight hayride, or picnicking in the woods near the infamous Dyer rock. The names of both Thomas Carbery Sr. and John Mattingly appear in Newtown parish account books of the period, with Carbery supplying beef and corn in 1798–1799. As would become a pattern in the small number of extant documents about John

Mattingly, the reference to his commercial dealing on December 3, 1804, says, "John Mattingly by Wheatly 1 g. brandy."[17]

In addition to the peculiar red fog that shrouded Ann and John's wedding day, the event was tinged by family sorrow. Ann's older brother, John Baptist Carbery, had died just one month before at age twenty-seven of an "indisposition . . . of short duration, and extremely malignant." Well-liked, "Jackey" was a gentleman of integrity, who left behind a young widow. This was the second brother Ann had lost in four years. Her youngest sibling, Ignatius Henry, the last of at least ten children born to his forty-two-year-old mother, had died in 1799 at age two. The very recent death of her oldest brother undoubtedly cast a pall over the wedding. Six years later, Ann would name her firstborn son after her brother John Baptist Carbery, namesake of their first ancestor in America.[18]

Ann and John's marriage took place during a time of great upheaval in St. Mary's County. Between 1790 and 1810, nearly 20 percent of the population left the county. Many headed to Kentucky, but the Carberys, along with Ann and John Mattingly, went to the Federal City, probably about 1805. The area of lower Newtown (now part of Leonardtown, where Moll Dyer had perished) was one of the areas in St. Mary's that experienced the steepest decline in population after 1800. Ann's wedding to John at age nineteen ended her childhood and young adult days in rural St. Mary's County. As was the custom, her family identity shifted away from the Carberys and she became known as "Mrs. Mattingly," the name she would carry until the end of her life. From the earliest days of their marriage, the couple likely began planning for a new life together in the Federal City, the national capital that had been established just three years before in 1800.[19]

The Federal City, 1800–1822

Southern Maryland's decline in population was exacerbated by the American Embargo Act of 1807, which closed U.S. ports to ships from around the globe in response to French and English restrictions on American exports. Ultimately, the embargo, which was a catastrophe for the China trade in places like Salem, Massachusetts, did great damage to American producers, such as the tobacco farmers of St. Mary's County, whose warehouses were overflowing with tobacco that they could not sell. As the economy worsened, Ann and John Mattingly moved to Washington, along with several members of Ann's family.[20]

In the Federal City, Thomas Carbery Sr. reportedly worked as a contractor furnishing heavy timbers for ceilings and floors used in the construction of public buildings. During this period, there was much building to be done in Washington. The city's main roads, according to William Janson, who arrived in 1804, were in terrible condition, filled with deep ruts, rocks, and even stumps of trees. He reported seeing "half-starved cattle browsing among the bushes [that] present a melancholy spectacle to the stranger. Quails and other birds are constantly shot within a hundred yards of the Capitol during the sitting of Congress." Another visitor, John Melish, reached the Federal City in October 1806 by stagecoach from the Bladensburg Road. When it stopped at Steele's Hotel, where he was staying, nearly opposite the Capitol, he was informed that he was in the center of the city, though there were no other buildings in view.[21]

The Irish poet and satirist Thomas Moore, in a poem first published in 1806, observed Washington's muddy dreariness and caricatured it this way:

> This famed metropolis, where Fancy sees
> Squares in morasses, obelisks in trees;
> Which travelling fools and gazetteers adorn
> With shrines unbuilt and heroes yet unborn,
> Though naught but wood and ***** they see
> Where streets should run and sages *ought* to be![22]

The building of Washington as the nation's capital, then, lay entirely ahead, and Moore's satire, perhaps unwittingly, contains a glimmering prediction of the city's future grandeur and significance. The Federal City to which Ann and John moved in 1805 was rough-hewn, but ready for growth.

For a couple from a rural county in southern Maryland, however, the new Capital City was not without its charms, and in the early days of their marriage, before the birth of their first child, Mary Susan, in 1806, John and Ann may have been able to appreciate some of the simple pleasures and amusements it offered. Orchards of cherry, apple, and peach trees and lush bushes of flowering laurel and fragrant honeysuckle grew throughout the capital. The city's rivers abounded with several varieties of fish and turtles. Boating and picnicking were popular pastimes, especially for young people. Excursion parties left for Arlington, Virginia, via the canal, and barges and flatboats could be chartered for the trip. Some could sail, but more often they were poled. In those days, the water was deep enough to cross over into Virginia, so rowing and yachting clubs launched their regattas from that point. John and Ann could enjoy a sweet baked at Havener's Bakery near City Spring, north of C Street, or drink from one of several excellent springs in the city, including a chalybeate mineral spring, near what is now Catholic University, that people visited for its alleged healing properties.[23]

The Mall of today, with its landscaped grounds and monuments, was then merely a cow pasture, used by everybody in common. Residents either kept a cow or got milk from a neighbor who did. Wood for construction came up the river in flat-bottomed boats steered into Tiber Creek, which flowed in from the river at Seventeenth Street. The wood business, in which Thomas Carbery Sr. was busily engaged, was primarily carried out along what is now B Street, from Seventeenth Street down to Sixth Street, and it prospered when the canal was extended to that point. At least twenty-four wood yards sprang up along the banks of the canal. Thomas Carbery Sr. built a federal-style home at 423 Sixth Street SE in 1803 in the Navy Yard section of town. This house was enlarged and ornate features were added later, but for its day, it was roomy and comfortable. At that time, the Navy Yard area, according to Madison Davis, was a neighborhood that had the "character of an English village," with a common, a skating pond, and fields for hunting and woods for collecting nuts. It is likely that Ann and John would have lived with her family on Sixth Street for some period when they first moved to the Capital City. They welcomed their daughter Mary

Susan on September 20, 1806, a day that began with fog but turned into a lovely autumn afternoon.[24]

The early years in Washington were a time of blessings and sorrows for Ann and John Mattingly. Fewer than three years after the birth of Susan, their son, John Baptist Carbery Mattingly, arrived on a stormy February 19, 1809. After another three years, John Mattingly's father, Barton Mattingly, died in early 1812, and on March 8 of that year, John was named as a beneficiary of Barton's will, which had been signed in Maryland in September 1807. A transcription error in which John's name is left off the property distribution has made it difficult for genealogists to trace John's lineage from Barton. John's name does not appear in copies of the distribution made for the court; the names of his stepmother, stepsister, siblings, niece, and nephew are listed. Barton Mattingly's entire estate was valued at $146.23. His widow, Jemima, took her widow's thirds, at $48.74. The daughter of Barton and Jemima, Pann, was given $12.18. The rest of the estate, $85.26, was divided by one-sixth to John's three siblings and Barton's two named grandchildren. Though John's name is not listed, his share of $14.21 is included in the total distribution.[25]

A few months after Barton Mattingly's death, Ann's father, Thomas Carbery Sr., also died, on July 12, 1812. A copy of his will has not been found, but Ann would likely have received a sum of money from his estate. It is not known when Ann and John were able to set up a home separate from the Carbery family on Sixth Street, but a couple of significant events in their lives might suggest a time frame of 1809–1813. Perhaps they established their own home after the birth of their second child in 1809, or possibly after Ann's inheritance in 1812–1813. John's inheritance of $14.21, about $200 today, would not have bought much. Where they lived in Washington before Ann moved back to her brother's home in 1815 is difficult to ascertain, because the District of Columbia census of 1810, along with other important records, was destroyed in 1814 when the British attacked the nation's capital.

During these emotionally tumultuous times for the family, Congress declared war against the British. On May 20, 1813, John Mattingly enrolled as a private in Major King's regiment in the District of Columbia militia under the command of Captain William McKee. He served approximately one month, until June 17, for which he was paid eight dollars. John reenlisted for two more months, until August 19, at the same rate of pay. But his military record has this curious notation: "Has been absent all the time." It is not known why John Mattingly served only one-third of his enlistment.[26]

During August 1814, the eight thousand residents of the Federal City sweltered under a brutal heat wave that contributed to swarms of pestilent mosquitoes in the city. With the oppressive weather and the scarcity of provisions, army morale was affected, and the city soon came under a full assault by the British. The problem of absences from the military was widespread enough to elicit this regimental order from Adjutant William McKenney on September 22, 1814: "In pursuance of brigade order, the commanding officers of companies will immediately furnish the adjutant with a correct list of all such persons who have absented themselves, *without leave,* from their respective companies, and who have so remained more than forty-eight hours, in order that they may be advertised as deserters, according to the law."[27]

Three days later, the army stepped up its efforts to enforce order in the troops, and the following notice appeared: "The officers commanding companies will, without delay, cause to be advertised in a newspaper of Washington or Georgetown, all such persons as have, *without leave,* absented themselves from their respective companies for more than forty-eight hours, offering a reward of $5 (five dollars) for any such absentee delivered to them in camp." John Mattingly's name does not appear to have been published, though he is clearly listed as absent without leave during his two months of service in 1813. Advertising for these AWOL soldiers in September 1814 came much too late, however; the month before, the City of Washington had come under attack by the British.[28]

The British had set their sights on Baltimore but clearly understood the psychological effect on Americans of decimating the Capital City of the new nation. As four thousand British troops marched in, most of the residents fled. It is likely that Ann would have evacuated the city with her two young children, Susan, nearly eight, and John, just five years old. On

August 24, American defenders were routed at the Battle of Bladensburg, and the city was left vulnerable. Dolley Madison famously fled the White House with a full-length portrait of George Washington under her arm that had been ripped from the walls of the president's house.

When the British general, Robert Ross, who was negotiating a truce with the Americans, was attacked by patriots in a house at the corner of Maryland Avenue, Constitution Avenue, and Second Street NE in Washington, D.C., the British became enraged. They killed everyone who had been in the house and burned it to the ground. The invaders went on to burn the Senate, the House of Representatives, the White House, the Library of Congress, and the U.S. Treasury Building, among other landmarks. It was during this attack that the census and other early records of the city were destroyed. Less than a day after the attacks began, they ended when a hurricane and tornado providentially passed through the city, scattering the invading troops and extinguishing the fires. The British had controlled Washington for only twenty-six hours. By 1815, the Treaty of Ghent ended the conflict, and Washington began to rebuild.

Against the background of these dramatic national events, John's difficulties began to intensify and affect his marriage. Sometime after 1805, when Ann and John relocated to Washington, John appears to have entered into a business arrangement with Ann's younger brother, Lewis Carbery, whose name appears with his in a court record. Other records show that John was buying vast amounts of supplies from the Washington Commercial Company, a general wholesale business begun in the city in 1808. According to company account books, presented as court evidence, by February 1814, John already was carrying a debt for purchases of large quantities of sugar, flour, coffee, bread, crackers, cigars, and whiskey. During the early years of the war, John may have been supplying American troops, but given his AWOL status in the militia during this same period, it is more likely he was either supplying ships in the busy port of Washington or selling to the various inns that the Nevitts on his mother's side of the family were operating in the city. John Mattingly may also have begun to show symptoms of a mysterious and debilitating illness that has plagued generations of Mattinglys and might account for his AWOL status and his mounting debt.[29]

The disease, which family members call the "creeping paralysis," has crippled the Mattinglys of southern Maryland for nearly 350 years. When Thomas Mattingly, John's ancestor, sailed from England to St. Mary's County, he carried in his genes a form of juvenile amyotrophic lateral sclerosis (ALS, also known as Lou Gehrig's disease). This nonfatal but devastating muscular disorder, now called ALS4, has been traced to a small region of chromosome 9. It has beset generations of Mattinglys and over time has become known simply as "the Mattingly disorder." The disease attacks the body's motor neurons, which connect muscles to the brain and the spinal cord. When the motor neurons die and the muscles are not engaged, they begin to deteriorate. Unlike typical ALS, the disease does not attack the respiratory system and throat, so sufferers can survive for many years. Weakness typically begins in the ankles and progresses to the arms, legs, and fingers and eventually moves to the neck. Descendents of Thomas Mattingly have a fifty-fifty chance of passing it to their offspring.

Symptoms of the disease may begin to appear as early as age two, although the average age of onset is seventeen. As children, sufferers are likely less athletic than their peers. When the disorder begins to manifest more obviously, in the late teens, one of the earliest signs is a stiff gait that affects walking. By age thirty or forty, the muscles of the legs and arms are wasted, and people with Mattingly disorder can no longer walk. The disease also destroys the padded muscle that most people have between their thumb and forefinger, which gives their hands a pincerlike look. Certainly, no one in the second decade of the nineteenth century would have had an understanding of this devastating genetic disease. The weakness would likely have been interpreted as laziness, and perhaps an unwillingness to work. It is not known how John Mattingly coped with his progressively decreasing capacities, but there are suggestions that he abused alcohol.[30]

In a court order issued the day before Ann and John's fourteenth wedding anniversary, November 8, 1817, the marshal of the District of Columbia ordered that John Mattingly, "late of Washington County," should appear in court to answer the charges against him. The documents filed with this order show John Mattingly owing John McGowan, a principal in the Washington Commercial Company, a staggering debt of $1078.72, plus $65.82 in interest—an enormous sum for the day, equal to $18,000 to $19,000 today. The debts date to before February 1814 and continue through June 23, 1815, for supplies such as flour, bread, and whiskey. During the siege of Washington in August 1814, Americans deliberately torched storehouses at the wharves of the Potomac to prevent arms and munitions from falling into the hands of the British invaders. It is possible that the supplies John Mattingly had purchased from the Washington Commercial Company went up in flames.

On December 30, 1814, a notice appeared in the *Washington Intelligencer* that John's brother, Thomas, had been imprisoned in the Washington jail for debt. He may have become involved with some of the unfortunate business failures of his brother, connected to the operation of local inns, and he, too, might have been afflicted with the creeping paralysis. Eight days before the British burned the city of Washington, on August 16, 1814, John had purchased two barrels of crackers at $9.68. Purchases of sundries, whiskey, and flour continued, according to the account book, until June 1815. John's business failures were likely a key factor in stress on his marriage because by 1815, Ann had moved with the children to her brother's house on Sixth Street. It is not known where John lived during this period. A dozen years after her wedding in the quaint little church in Newtown, Ann's life shifted away from her husband and back toward the Carberys.

Much of the Carbery prominence and prosperity was still to come, yet even by 1815, they were well established in Washington. Shortly after the war had ended, Captain Thomas Carbery erected Carbery's Wharf near the recently completed Washington City Canal. Passenger steamers from Alexandria, Virginia, unloaded there, and materials to rebuild the city after the war's destruction were ferried through the wharf. This profitable business would be the foundation of the large fortune that Thomas Carbery would accumulate during his lifetime.[31]

There is no evidence that John lived with his family in the household

of Thomas Carbery beginning in 1815, and John's whereabouts are not documented after Ann's move to her brother's home. After the notation in the
Washington Commercial Company records in June of that year, no mention
of him surfaces again until December 1817, when he was summoned to appear in court. Judge Brent commanded the marshal to take "John Mattingly,
late of Washington County if he shall be found within the county of Washington, in your said district, and him safely keep, so that you have his body
before the Circuit Court of the district of Columbia, to be held for the county
aforesaid, at the city of Washington, on the fourth Monday of December
next, to answer unto John McGowan on a plea of trespass on the case and
so forth."[32] We will probably never know whether Ann knew John's whereabouts during 1815–1817. When she discovered the lump in her breast in 1817,
it was the Carbery family, not her husband, who rallied to support her.

John's court appearance did not take place until June 10, 1819. Given
that he was summoned to court two years before he appeared, he was probably incarcerated in debtor's prison from December 1817 until June 1819, as
laws at the time were harsh, and one could be jailed for a debt of less than
a dollar. Even prominent citizens were not immune to imprisonment, and
documents relating to jails of the period suggest that many respectable
family men were put in prison for extended periods. While John remained
incarcerated, Thomas Carbery moved with Ann, her two children, and
other family members in 1818 into a brand new Federal-style brick house he
had built on the corner of C and Seventeenth Streets. It had "several unusual
features for a Washington Federal house. The siding of the gable roof had
no molding but was flush with the side brick walls, and the entrance opened
to the side rather than on the main façade."[33]

Foggy Bottom was also a more upscale neighborhood than the home
on Sixth Street near the Navy Yard. By moving to a prestigious neighborhood, very close to the White House and near John Van Ness, the prominent
founder of the bank where Thomas worked, the Carberys were stepping up
in the social hierarchy. Their parish, St. Patrick's, was the spiritual home of
long-established and wealthy Catholic families. Ann and her children lived
in this house with the family slaves, her sisters, her widowed sister-in-law,

and possibly her mother, who passed away at age sixty-two on January 2, 1819, in Washington. But as the family settled into the new house, Ann's health worsened, and she was increasingly confined to her bed.

John Mattingly was not alone in having financial troubles during this period. Early in 1819, while he awaited trial, the nation was plunged into a period of economic distress. After the War of 1812, there was, as historian Constance McLaughlin Green notes, a "nation-wide orgy of speculation" driven by dubious paper money. Early in 1819, these inflated values began to collapse. Green offers the following example: "A wharf and storehouses purchased two or three years before for $17,000 brought $1,200," only 7 percent of its original value. Commerce dwindled, commodity prices shrank, real estate values plummeted, and credit was nearly impossible to obtain. In the midst of this depression, banks began to fail and became the target of accusations of greed and fraud. John's debt had been accumulated during the inflationary boom years, and paying it off became more and more difficult.[34]

Both the Carberys and John's brother, Stephen, who lived near the Carberys in affluent Ward 1 of the city in 1820, had a comfortable standard of living for the time. Stephen's household had six free blacks living with his family of five, consisting of himself, his wife, and three daughters. It is reasonable to assume that John's probable incarceration was something of an embarrassment for both the Carbery family and for his brother. We may never know what John did to make him become such a pariah that neither side of the family was willing to bail him out of jail.[35]

In 1820, Thomas Carbery was serving as a city official and president of the National Metropolitan Bank, one of the largest financial institutions in Washington. The bank underwrote the army payroll during the War of 1812 and about 20 percent of the reconstruction of federal buildings after the war, including the Capitol and the White House. That year, the household of Thomas Carbery consisted of eleven people: twenty-nine-year-old Thomas; his sisters Ruth, Catharine, and thirty-six-year-old Ann Mattingly; Ann's two children, Susan, age fourteen, and John, age eleven; and five slaves, two males and three females.[36]

In early 1821, a John Mattingly attended meetings of the Union Fire Company with Thomas Carbery. Because Ann's husband John was still likely incarcerated at this time, the mention of a John Mattingly at these meetings suggests it was their twelve-year-old son attending with his uncle. According to the *National Intelligencer,* that year Thomas Carbery was named as an engineer and John Mattingly as a hoseman. The following year, the same paper lists Thomas Carbery and J. Mattingly as hosemen. In these days, fire companies were composed of volunteers, and many of the men in the Union Fire Company were highly respected citizens. Thomas may have wished to mentor young John and act as a surrogate father to the boy. At the volunteer fire company meetings, young John would have had the opportunity to associate with many community leaders.[37]

During the week of October 28, 1822, the following notice appeared Monday through Thursday in the *National Intelligencer,* announcing that John Mattingly was seeking legal relief from his imprisonment for debt:

> Washington County, District of Columbia
>
> On the petition of John Mattingly, an insolvent debtor, confined in the prison of Washington County for debt: Notice is hereby given to the creditors of the said John Mattingly, that, on the first Monday of November next, at 11 o'clock at the court room . . . "An Act for the relief of insolvent debtors within the District of Columbia" will be administered to the said insolvent, and a trustee appointed for the benefit of the creditors, unless sufficient cause to the contrary be then and there shewn.
>
> . . . And it is further ordered that the petitioner . . . appear at the time and place, for the purpose aforesaid.

According to the act mentioned, passed in the District of Columbia during 1802, John Mattingly could have been freed from prison to begin to work off his debt. His long-awaited court date was set for Monday, November 4, 1822, though his appearance would be moved up by a few days for unknown reasons.[38]

While John remained confined to jail, his brother-in-law's fortunes continued to rise. Thomas Carbery had served admirably during the War of 1812 and had become a captain in the militia. The title pleased him, and throughout his life Thomas continued to be called Captain Carbery. From 1819 to 1821, he served as a two-term city counselor and a bank official. Despite the economic downturn, while Carbery was in office, the city of Washington had passed a new charter that took effect on May 15, 1820. Among the changes enacted were the creation of a board of health and the development of a building code. Thomas helped forge a progressive agenda for improving the Capital City.[39]

The Carbery family was noted for its generosity to the poor, especially orphans, and also for its deeply religious Catholicism. Not only had their aunt Elizabeth been the first professed nun in the United States, but Thomas and Ann's oldest sister was a Carmelite, and their younger brother Joseph had become a Jesuit priest. In 1822, Captain Thomas Carbery paid a visit to Joseph, stationed at St. Inigoes parish in St. Mary's County. Gazing down the St. Mary's River, Thomas and Joseph discussed the historic founding of the American Catholic community on its banks, and Joseph mentioned that the original cannons from the *Ark* and the *Dove* lay in the mud and silt just below the waterline. Thomas, motivated by his family connections to the history of St. Mary's County and by his love for his home state of Maryland, vowed to spare no expense in retrieving the cannons from the destructive salty tidal water. The cannons were a link not only to the Bretton family, but to the Mattingly progenitor, Thomas Mattingly, and other old-line Maryland families.

According to Edith Marden Ridout, a historian for the Daughters of the American Revolution, the captain waited until ebb tide "when the water was but two and a half feet deep, by digging away the sand in two places and placing two heavy timber chains beneath one of the large cannon, and passing the chains over strong beams supported on two scows, he found that flood tide raised the scows sufficiently to drag the gun from the bed of the river. The scows were then pushed near shore, and the cannon hauled one by one by a timber cart up in front of the old St. Inigoes Mansion, where they remained many years." In 1840, the Reverend Joseph Carbery presented two of the cannons as a gift to the state of Maryland, where they were displayed in the entrance hall of the State House in Annapolis. In 1908, the Daughters of the American Revolution placed a plaque on them that says: "This cannon was brought from England by the First Settlers, March 5, 1634. Mounted on the Walls of the Fort at Old St. Mary's. Recovered From the St. Mary's River, 1822. Presented to the State in 1840, by Rev. Joseph Carbery. This Tablet is Placed by the Peggy Stewart Tea Party Chapter, Daughters of the American Revolution, of Annapolis, Maryland, 'Maryland Day,' March 25, 1908." Two other cannons were on display at Georgetown University for many years. Members of the Carbery family took enormous pride in their connections to the Catholic founders of Maryland, and one can imagine Ann Mattingly in her sickbed, enjoying her brother's story of recovering the old artillery that helped protect the family of her esteemed ancestor, William Bretton, during his settlement days in St. Mary's County.[40]

During this eventful year for the family, Ann's uncle Henry, a well-known hero of the American Revolution, died on May 26, 1822. Henry Carbery survived a wound in his side where a British musket ball lodged during the war; it could not be removed and caused him pain for the rest of his life. Despite his war injury, he served with distinction during the War of 1812. Ann had been very close to her uncle and his wife, Sybilla. The laudatory eulogy of Henry Carbery in the *National Intelligencer* is in marked contrast to the silence that would surround the death of her husband six months later. Henry Carbery was praised as a passionate philanthropist, with "fascinating" manners and "inflexible integrity." Though it would later be revealed in probate records that he, too, died insolvent, his reputation remained untarnished.[41]

During 1822, Ann remained gravely ill in her brother's home and under the care of her two unmarried sisters, Ruth and Catharine Carbery, and their slaves. She was nearly a recluse, living vicariously through the activities of the respected men in her family—her prominent brother, Thomas, and her devout brother, Joseph, who was performing such good work at St. Inigoes. Her sixteen-year-old daughter, Susan, also helped care for her.

Her son, John Baptist Carbery Mattingly, was now thirteen. He was quick, alert, and growing to be very handsome. Secretly, though, his mother may have worried that young John seemed to resemble not so much her adored Carbery brothers, but his father, who had turned out to be a disappointment to so many. During the early period of their marriage, there had likely been a painful tug-of-war in her heart between her affections for her husband and a growing awareness of the gap between the abilities and integrity of the Carberys and his. But now, all affection seemed to be lost. In the effusive eulogies for her uncle, and the political ambitions of her brother, Ann must have been even more keenly aware of these contrasts. She likely hoped and prayed that her son could cultivate the good traits he inherited from the Carbery side.

Less than a month after the death of Henry Carbery, Thomas narrowly won election as mayor of Washington, D.C. Even though one of his opponents, Roger Weightman, had the support of the powerful *National Intelligencer,* Captain Carbery prevailed. On June 4, 1822, the results were announced. Carbery had garnered 314 votes, Weightman, 258, and his other two opponents 101 and 56 votes, respectively. A writer in the *Metropolitan and Georgetown National Messenger* observed, "The election being contested with so much spirit and the rival parties each marshaling their forces with such uncommon ardor, proved that a great degree of popularity must have been requisite to have assured either of the triumph." Carbery's victory was later challenged on the basis that propertyless voters in two wards had cast their votes for him, during a period when the electorate was limited by the charter of 1820 "to white males who had paid at least fifty cents in taxes and had resided in the city for a year." Even the impoverished John Mattingly could have voted in the election, had he not been in debtor's prison.[42]

Carbery, then, still mourning his illustrious uncle, became "the poor man's successful candidate," who, as soon as the court decision seated him, "enrolled in the assessment books the names of men who, according to outraged conservatives, owned no property but their clothes." On January 9, 1823, Weightman won his challenge to the election when a court decided that it had been illegally conducted and the result was therefore

void. Carbery, however, remained in office, since his term would expire
in June 1824, and the court proceedings to remove him could not be completed before then. From her confinement in the mayor's home, Ann likely
awaited news with the rest of the family of the dramatic events following
the election. On good days, when she could join the others for dinner or
sit with the family in the parlor, she perhaps marveled at the complicated
and mercurial world of men and wondered how young John would fare in
it when he grew to be a man.[43]

Captain Carbery thoroughly enjoyed his hard-won prominent position, hosting dinners and formalizing the celebration of the Fourth of July in
the nation's capital. As chairman of the event, he organized an elegant dinner at Strother's Hotel in the city, which several prominent citizens, government officials, and foreign dignitaries attended. Under his administration,
the first Washington directory was published. The city began collecting
statistics on population and disease and continued to improve its streets and
water supply. A town meeting style of government gave opinions on national
issues directly to Congress, so the sphere of local government was extended
during the early days of Washington, D.C., with resolutions being passed
on international events as far away as Greece. Carbery played a key role in
insisting that residents of the Federal City could vote in national elections,
a privilege that had not yet been secured at this time. Thomas Carbery was
active in helping to found the Washington Female Orphan Asylum and
passed progressive legislation relating to the situation of debtors in the city.[44]

The Carbery family, then, descended from genteel planters and important founders of colonial Maryland, produced two men, Henry and
Thomas, who served with distinction in two key national wars and rose
to positions of prominence in the new Federal City. In 1803, Ann Carbery
Mattingly had married into the less financially successful Mattingly family.
Instead of being a military hero, John was a deserter. Instead of becoming
a successful businessman, as did Thomas and her other brothers, Lewis
and James, John Mattingly made bad investments and lost money. When
Ann moved into her brother's household in 1815, the marriage of a dozen
years had apparently run its course. The debts on John McGowan's balance

sheet included large quantities of whiskey, so perhaps John Mattingly had developed habits that his wife found insupportable. Given Ann's Catholicism, divorce was out of the question, so separation may have seemed a more respectable solution.

While the lowly citizens of Washington helped elect Ann's brother Thomas, while her uncle was lionized for his generosity to the poor, and while Ann's health continued to worsen, John Mattingly lingered in the horrendous conditions inside the Washington jail. Both Ann and John now suffered parallel confinements—hers because of illness, his in a prison house packed with the insane, escaped slaves, criminals, and insolvent debtors. A series of reports detailing the condition of the Washington jail during 1818–1819 tell a story of hopelessness, as debtors like John Mattingly could be held for years awaiting a court appearance. A committee led by future mayor and Carbery political opponent Samuel Smallwood filed a report that noted, among other things, "Prisoners said their allowance of food was generally too scant and the quality generally bad." The two-story jail was arranged so that the worst criminals were downstairs; as a debtor, John Mattingly likely would have been confined upstairs.[45]

Reports describe the building as defective and "totally unfit . . . for the purpose for which it is occupied," with prisoners existing in "miserable wretched conditions." A summary report called the jail "destructive to the health of its tenants, incompetent for their safe-keeping, and an annoyance to the neighbourhood." In spring 1818, a group of physicians asked to inspect the jail made special note in their report of the condition of the debtors' apartments, writing: "these rooms did not exhibit that appearance of cleanliness and comfort which we were prepared to expect; on the contrary, [they] were in a filthy and neglected state; in addition to which, the prisoners complained of being neglected, and of a want of a proper diet. When we consider that these unhappy persons are frequently thrown into confinement from unavoidable misfortune and that the most deserving men in the community are sometimes reduced to the same degraded state [of] wretchedness from similar causes; we are compelled by justice, and humanity, to recommend toward them a different mode of treatment."[46]

The report notes that criminals slept on damp stone floors and were covered only with a filthy blanket. The investigating committee recommended that prison rooms be "white-washed with good lime, at least once a month; and during winter season, one or two stoves" be provided. The physicians were especially concerned about an open putrefying "common sewer" that contaminated the air of the jail and concluded, "The present establishment is wholly inadequate for the security of Criminals or the comfort of unfortunate Debtors." In January 1819 another report was issued, noting some improvements that had taken place following the recommendation of the physicians the previous May. A more compassionate jailer had been hired, one who did his best to make the prisoners as comfortable as possible. Stoves to provide heat had been added, but they malfunctioned and the furniture and the prisoners were now covered in soot. The common sewer where human waste collected beneath the jail continued to produce "a putrid exhalation which is poisonous to the health of the prisoners." Several of the prisoners had contracted dysentery during the previous fall, and the investigator attested to the prisoners having a "cadaverous appearance . . . from some secret cause." He also noted that the clothes of some of the prisoners were "covered with vermin."[47]

On October 26, 1822, a few days earlier than his scheduled court date, John Mattingly appeared and pleaded for release under the Act for the Relief of Insolvent Debtors. Mayor Thomas Carbery was the signing justice of the peace who appeared with John to verify that Ann's husband had no real property but the clothes on his back. The five creditors listed were from Georgetown, including Francis Lowndes, who owned some warehouses on the Georgetown wharf. John Mattingly did not sign his name on the document but made an X in a shaky hand. He was released from prison that day. It is not known whether he returned to Georgetown to the living quarters described in the census or came under the care of Thomas Carbery. According to material in private family archives, John Mattingly died fewer than four weeks later on November 30, 1822, a day of rain in the morning, followed by afternoon sunshine. He was one of the 157 adults who died in the city during that year. The death records for this period are published

John Mattingly's palsied "X" as his signature in 1822, from insolvent debtors' case files. Courtesy of the National Archives and Records Administration.

as composites, so we do not know the exact cause of John's death, but there were five suicides among them, and five died of intemperance.[48]

The death of Ann's husband John, likely in midlife, and the ensuing early death of his and Ann's son John Baptist Carbery Mattingly at age thirty-nine suggests a possibility that goes beyond compiled statistical lists. The X mark in John Mattingly's hand on the court papers of October 1822 is an intriguing clue. We know Ann Mattingly was literate, and notes in Rev. Stephen Dubuisson's hand refer to her quick and lively mind. So she probably would have married a man who could read and write. But, perhaps a victim of the mysterious and debilitating creeping paralysis, by the time he was released from jail, John could manage to write only that palsied X on the court papers with a cramped and pincerlike hand.

The documentation of John Mattingly's death in family papers is corroborated by an affidavit labeled "Washington City, 15th March, 1823" that
states "Mrs. Mattingly . . . is now a widow, having lost her husband but a
few months since." No notice of his death or burial records have surfaced.
Archival material indicates that Ann was, by this point, too ill or too distanced from her estranged husband to attend his funeral. John Mattingly
came to an untimely end, with the days leading up to his death spent in a
cold stone cell, recalling Moll Dyer's solitary death in the frozen Maryland
woods a century and a quarter before.[49]

Did the curse of Moll Dyer, a legend from colonial Maryland that the
old-line families might have passed from generation to generation, somehow
extend to Ann? Perhaps so. At age thirty-eight, she was a widow, the des-
ignation now the only remnant of a long-broken marriage. And though her
status as widow was certainly more respectable than that of estranged wife,
she was also suffering from a deadly and debilitating illness. At the same
time, she was viewed by others as a model of Christian fortitude, and her
family connections in religious orders gave her access to a powerful network
of prayer. In seeming defiance of Moll Dyer's curse or other superstitious
explanations for the trials of her life, Ann Mattingly was now poised to receive an extraordinary blessing. Prince Hohenlohe's most famous American
miracle would soon change Ann's Mattingly's world—and help define the
place of Catholicism in the United States.

FOUR

Thaumaturgus and Priest

A miracle becomes a proof of the character, or doctrine,
of him by whom it was wrought.

—Timothy Dwight, *Theology, Explained and Defended* (1819)

Ellwangen, Germany, October 1777

The sixteen-year-old girl, her arms pinned tight by her mother and brothers, was pulled into the room, a tiny cell in the back part of the former Benedictine Monastery of Ellwangen. The Romanesque church is dedicated to St. Vitus, whose passionate worship in the Middle Ages led to such frenetic dancing before his statue that his name became associated with an abnormal involuntary movement disorder called *Chorea sancti viti,* or St. Vitus's dance. The young girl's pupils went dark with fear as her family pushed her into the straight-backed wooden chair in the center of the room. There her mother held her forcibly in front of a small table where the black-gowned priest sat with a silver crucifix in his hand. Light filtered in from high windows cut into the thick walls of the cell, and the air was dense with tension and the smell of candle smoke. The priest, Rev. Johann Joseph Gassner, began speaking to the girl softly in German, explaining the procedure that was about to take place. When the girl nodded her understanding, Gassner, loudly and in Latin now, commanded the demons that possessed her to inflict their utmost pain.

The girl squirmed in her mother's arms, groaning and growling as if she were being viciously prodded and poked. As the violence of her struggles increased, her brothers stepped forward to restrain her even more forcefully, and her mother burst into tears. The girl's groans escalated until they were deep and guttural, no longer sounding human and as if issuing from the wellspring of her soul. Then she lashed out at the priest in a voice

81

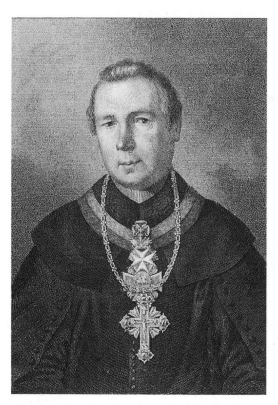

Prince Alexander
Hohenlohe's portrait
from his memoir
*Lichtblicke und
Erlebnisse aus
der Welt und dem
Priesterleben;
gesammelt in den
Jahren 1815–1833*
(1836).

that seemed alien and masculine, spitting out profanity and blasphemous words against God. The priest ordered the demons to give the girl an attack of epilepsy. Her brothers stepped back, and she collapsed on the floor, saliva bubbling from her mouth. While her stunned family watched her flailing, the priest commanded in a loud voice, "Cessit!" the Latin word for "let it cease." Having demonstrated to the girl, to her family, and to himself that this was a case of demonic possession, Gassner, with the full approval of the young girl, began an exorcism to expel her demons.

In the valley of the winding Jagst River, nestled near some of the most ancient forests in southern Germany, the charming medieval town of Ell-wangen once again seemed to be under vicious assault by the devil. About two hundred years before, some of Germany's most intense witch hunts had happened here, resulting in the execution at the beginning of the seventeenth century of about 450 people. Now, in late-eighteenth-century Ellwangen, a spate of demonic possessions had gripped the town. Johann Joseph Gassner rose to fame as uniquely gifted to wrestle down the devil. In October 1777, Gassner performed hundreds of exorcisms in Ellwangen alone, defying direct orders from his emperor and Pope Pius VI to halt the practice.[1]

One of Gassner's staunchest and most passionate patrons was Karl Albrecht, prince of Hohenlohe and Waldenburg, whose son Alexander would, in the next generation, arise to fame because of his own alleged miraculous healing powers. Prince Karl had been long fascinated with exorcism and was one of several noblemen and noblewomen who signed affidavits attesting that they had witnessed 232 successful exorcisms performed by Gassner in Ellwangen during a single month in 1777. The short, plump, clean-shaven Gassner, whose mild appearance in portraits belies the ferocity with which he did battle with the Prince of Evil, reportedly cured epileptics, cripples, and the blind using controversial and unconventional methods, including stroking and yanking on the limbs of those he was trying to cleanse.

When a sick person was seated before him, Gassner began with an *exorcismus probativus*, or test exorcism, in which, to determine whether the ailment was caused by a demon, he would instruct the evil spirit in Latin to perform certain acts. The demon, if it was present, according to historian H. C. Erik Midelfort, would move "around in the body and . . . evoke a wide range of horrible symptoms: swelling first here, and then there, fevers, headache, cramps, convulsions, tremors, and pains in one foot, then in the other." Once the presence of the demon was verified, Gassner continued to call on it to manifest itself in the patient's body, so that both he and the patient understood that the disease did not have a natural cause—a process Gassner called *praecepta*, precepts, or lessons. When the evidence was clear to both priest and patient that the illness was originating in a demonic possession, Gassner would perform an *exorcismus lenitivus*, a soothing exorcism, or if necessary, the more powerful *exorcismus expulsivus*, expelling exorcism, that would rid the patient of the devil.[2]

Like his successor, Alexander Hohenlohe, Gassner had more success curing women than men. His method of stroking his victims in their
affected areas, including the breasts and genitals, made him a target for accusations of scandal. Gassner enjoyed the full support of Alexander's father,
who worked to have the papal ban on his exorcisms lifted until the priest's
death in 1779, fifteen years before Alexander's birth. Even after Gassner's
death, Prince Karl continued to dabble in exorcisms and the supernatural.
In 1774, Gassner had published a little guide whose title is translated *Useful
Instruction in Fighting the Devil.* This tract caught the attention of Prince
Alexander Hohenlohe's future healing partner, the farmer Martin Michel,
who read Gassner's writings extensively. The life and work of Johann Gassner influenced both Alexander's father and the man who would join him
in the sensational healing of Princess Mathilde in 1821. By extension, it
influenced the prince who healed Mrs. Ann Mattingly.[3]

The end of Gassner's era was an important turning point in the history of the German confederation on two fronts: changes to the medical
system in the German states began in 1799 and concluded in 1807–1808 with
the *Organischen Edikt* (Organic Edict). This edict summarized and codi-
fied almost ten years of changes to the medical field in the German states,
essentially limiting the freedom of lay practitioners and professionalizing
the field of medicine. At the turn of the nineteenth century, the Catholic
Church in Bavaria had lost a number of its properties, including churches,
abbeys, and cloisters, because of secularization. It was also weakened by the
prominence of rationalism in Germany and recent prohibitions of church
traditions such as pilgrimages and Christmas decorations.[4]

While these restrictions were being imposed, an edict establishing parity between Catholics and Protestants was issued, culminating in
changes to the Bavarian constitution in 1818. It was in this charged arena
that Prince Hohenlohe's miracles were seen as a throwback to some of the
earlier folk traditions that Bavarian officials were trying to move away from.
Protestants especially were concerned about the prince's claims that the
Catholic Church was the one true church. Thus, Protestants were an as-
cending minority in Bavaria at this time; and in Washington, D.C., the Ho-

henlohe miracles came at a time when minority Catholics in North America were poised to lose some of their power and authority.[5]

Leopold Alexander Franz Emerich von Hohenlohe-Waldenburg-Schillingsfürst, was of noble lineage, born August 17, 1794, near what is now Württemberg. The family history of this polynomial young man stretched back to an eminent sixth-century progenitor, Arnulf of Metz (582–640), a Frankish nobleman who became first a consecrated bishop and then a saint. Alexander's direct ancestors included the Emperor Charlemagne, who had died at the beginning of the ninth century, and Prince Eberhard von Franken, whose brother Konrad was king of Germany from 911 to 918. Baron Ludwig Gustav von Hohenlohe-Schillingsfürst, Prince Alexander's great-great-great-grandfather, was the first von Hohenlohe to turn away from the Reformation and return to Catholicism in 1667. By the mid-eighteenth century, the family line had subdivided into a Protestant branch (Hohenlohe-Neuenstein) and a Catholic (Hohenlohe-Waldenburg). The latter branch further split into the houses Bartenstein and Schillingsfürst. In 1744, Holy Roman Emperor Charles VII Albert named the Hohenlohes Prince of the Holy Roman Empire. In 1757, thirty-seven years before the birth of Prince Alexander, Emperor Franz I elevated the Catholic branches to a princedom. Alexander's father, Karl Albrecht, became the reigning Prince of Schillingsfürst.[6]

The day after Alexander was born, his uncle, Prince Franz Karl von Hohenlohe, dean of the church of Ellwangen and general vicar and titular bishop of Tempe, baptized him in the family castle. His godfather, Archduke Leopold Alexander Joseph, a Hungarian palatine, a position similar to that of prime minister, was apparently unable to attend. Alexander was the last child of second marriages for both parents. Before his parents' marriage on August 15, 1773, Alexander's father, Karl Albrecht II, Royal General Major and Prince of Schillingsfürst, had two sons from his first marriage with Leopoldine, Princess of Loewenstein. She died in 1765, and both her children had died before their first birthdays. Alexander's Hungarian mother, Judith Freiin Reviczky von Recisnye, anglicized as Judith Rewitsky, had one son,

Emerich, from her first marriage with a Hungarian knight who had died. Alexander's father had served as an officer in the Austrian army and while stationed in Grosswardein, met the young widow and married her. His father, Prince Albrecht I, did not accept the young wife of his first son as one who befitted their rank. He tried to persuade the emperor to change the succession and humiliated his son in front of the emperor, accusing Prince Karl Albrecht of extravagant spending habits. His father's disapproval undoubtedly added stress to Karl Albrecht's emotional fragility, which manifested in part as an obsession with exorcism and other ritual practices.[7]

By the time of Alexander's birth his father had suffered a serious mental breakdown. He died on June 14, 1796, before Alexander, the last of his eighteen children, had turned two years old. Alexander formed an intense bond with his mother, Baroness Judith Rewitsky. She assumed the responsibility of raising the boy and would remain a central figure throughout his life. Alexander's mother had destined him from birth for the priesthood, and she was his first teacher in religious principles. Later, she engaged a French priest as his tutor, a former Jesuit, Rev. Riel. The prince's connection with exiled Jesuits and French émigrés would continue during the 1820s in Washington, D.C., as the Jesuits championed him in North America.[8]

Alexander was born during the height of France's postrevolution Reign of Terror, which was characterized by a wave of executions of presumed enemies of the state. The backdrop of a war-torn European continent shaped his youngest years. His older brothers had enlisted in the Austrian Army, which, joining with the forces of Prussia, Great Britain, Spain, Holland, and other nations, was defending the country's borders against the French Republic. He was just six years old when his brother Prince Albert Conrad died at Marengo, Italy, in a battle against the invading French, and was eleven when another brother, Prince Joseph, was killed in the rout of the Austrian Army by advancing Napoleonic troops at Ulm.

His childhood and teenage years were lived out during a period of great upheaval throughout Europe and in southern Germany. German culture had become increasingly secularized. Composed of a collection of states and principalities, German-speaking Europe was culturally and militarily dominated by Austria and Prussia. This was, of course, until Napoleon's victories forced some and enticed other German states into an alliance with the growing French Empire; these alliances were further strengthened by the union of Napoleon with the Austrian Archduchess Marie Louise, daughter of the emperor. Princes and nobility of German states defeated by Napoleon were degraded to the role of the French emperor's servants, and several German regions were entirely reorganized.

In May 1814, Pope Pius VII returned to Rome after five years of imprisonment under Napoleon, and this event sparked a resurgence in Catholicism. Just a month before the Pope's liberation, Napoleon's empire had fallen before a coalition of Austria, Russia, Prussia, and Britain. Once Napoleon had been removed from his throne, Europe's leaders turned their attention to the problem of restoring order throughout the continent. Meeting at the Congress of Vienna in 1814 and 1815, the leaders, led by Austria's Prince Klemens von Metternich, focused on the German lands. Reestablishing thirty-three German states, the Congress of Vienna then linked them loosely in a confederation that was designed to ensure the individual state's internal and external security. The congress also strengthened the position of the Catholic Church under the guidance of Cardinal Ercole Consalvi, but by 1817, theological debates and sectarian differences again began to predominate throughout the region.

One of his biographers, G. N. Pachtler, has characterized Alexander as an extremely sensitive, quiet, and introverted boy, but accounts of his boyhood vary wildly, underscoring the wide range of people's responses to him. Ludwig Sebastian, the most reliable of the early biographers, reports that Alexander loved to play war games, lost his books, and left his clothes in tatters and that he was disorganized, hard to control, and a habitual liar. His teachers praised his intellectual gifts yet bemoaned his lack of perseverance. Alexander's typical approach to his schoolwork was to begin a task at the last possible moment and then hurry to complete it. He was a prankster and relished undertaking dangerous physical challenges. Yet, from an early age, he showed a marked preference for the spiritual. One

Christmas morning, when both a toy horse and a toy altar were under the tree for Alexander, he surprised and pleased his mother by ignoring the horse and making a dash for the altar.[9]

The sense of entitlement that his thousand-year-old noble name conferred upon him may have contributed to the mediocre academic performance that marked his school years. In October 1804, at age ten, he was admitted to the Collegium Theresianum, an elite school that had been founded in Vienna by Jesuits in 1746. Its mission was to educate young royalty, who would be expected to follow their preliminary studies at the school with two additional years of education in philosophy and then three additional years in the study of law. Following the turmoil resulting from the suppression of the Jesuits, the collegium temporarily closed its doors in 1783, but Emperor Franz I reopened it in 1797 as the Theresianum Knight Academy. The Knight Academy, until its closing in 1848, offered elementary education that prepared students for the university as well as for the study of philosophy and law.

After four years at the Theresianum, the young prince began to weary of its military atmosphere and transferred in 1808 to the Academic Gymnasium in Bern, Switzerland, a Latin school with six grades where he studied Latin, Greek, and French. But two years later, the school's strict rules prompted him to withdraw and return to the Theresianum in Vienna. Following another year at that institution, seventeen-year-old Alexander, with special permission and funding given to him by Emperor Franz I, fulfilled his mother's fondest wish and entered the seminary to begin studies for the priesthood. Alexander chafed at the meager allowance the emperor had set for him, however, and complained that he did not have enough money to afford breakfast or a sandwich, to partake of afternoon tea or wine with his meals, or to buy writing paper or gloves. Franz I replied that for Alexander to have such luxuries would place him above the lifestyle affordable to the other students in the seminary. This nobleman, then, was an unlikely saint for Catholics in an American nation dedicated to democratic principles.[10]

On September 8, 1812, at the age of eighteen and on his mother's birthday, Prince Alexander gave his first public sermon at the estate of his brother-in-law, Earl Fries von Lengbach. Alexander's sister praised his performance. A progress report on the young prince, sent to his benefactor, noted that he was a good student whose behavior was above reproach. But the Austrian papal nuncio, or envoy, Antonio Severoli, strongly criticized Alexander's performance as a student, writing: "I say this much for his capability: with quite mediocre talent he has completed his course of study. With much irregularity and countless interruptions, nothing has been completed, and the end result stands at little more than nothing."[11]

In the fall of 1813, Alexander transferred to the Hungarian seminary for priests in Tyrnau. From the new school, he mailed an extremely critical letter complaining about Bishop Sigismund Anton, Baron von Hohenwart, the head of the seminary in Vienna. The prince charged that, under Hohenwart's leadership, the teachings of the Pope were being ignored and that the truths of Catholicism were not being taught. He also noted that the reason his debts were accumulating was because he was giving alms to the poor. Hohenwart responded to his pupil's attack with a stinging reprimand. He reminded Alexander of the many seminary rules he had broken and accused him of getting himself in debt and of neglecting his studies. The chastened prince wrote an apology and begged his former teacher's forgiveness. With this apology, the emperor restored Alexander's allowance.[12]

Ten years before his miraculous cure of Ann Mattingly caused a sensation in the United States, in March 1814, even before his ordination, the twenty-year-old Hohenlohe was promised a position in Olmütz. That fall, he left the seminary in Tyrnau and transferred to the University of Ellwangen to finish his studies. He lived with his uncle, Franz Karl von Hohenlohe-Schillingsfürst, pastor of Ellwangen, who had baptized him. According to one historian, in April 1815, the prince requested a special favor from the Vatican to be ordained early. Severoli issued a harsh denial, stating that the prince's behavior and principles did not merit such an action; if he could not change, he should not enter the priesthood. Severoli warned Prince Hohenlohe against overarching ambition, worldly desires, and the temptation to drink too much wine.[13]

The Vatican did not grant a favor, and Alexander was ordained in

September 18, 1815, at the age of twenty-one by his uncle. The well-known
professor of theology and future bishop of Ratisbon, Johann Michael Sailer,
gave the sermon at his ordination. Disgusted, the nuncio wrote to Rome
that "the bad priest's behavior is to be observed and he is to be prevented
from becoming a bishop." His only talents, he added, were "impertinence
and cant." Severoli also continued his condemnation of the prince, calling
him a "notorious liar, and a profligate."[14]

Hohenlohe's first experience in pastoral care was in Schillingsfürst.
From his earliest days in the priesthood, Alexander, like his father, was
intrigued with exorcisms and practices of spiritual healing. Rumors spread
that the young priest was able to cast out devils. One day during the absence
of the Franciscan pastor he was assisting, he attempted to exorcise a Protestant woman who came to him from Württemberg. In the commotion that
followed this, the strange woman had to be expelled from the town. Civil
authorities censored him for causing the disturbance, and religious authorities ordered him to study and follow diocesan regulations. The prince seems
to have moderated his activities and is reported to have ably ministered to
the sick during a typhus epidemic in Schillingsfürst the following year.[15]

In March 1816, Hohenlohe was accepted into the Order of Malta, the
same year this ancient order established its headquarters in Rome after the
Napoleonic Wars, and he affiliated himself with the Society of the Sacred
Heart, which had kept alive the spirit of the Society of Jesus, the Jesuits,
during the suppression. The prince traveled to Munich, where he was introduced to the king of Bavaria, Maximilian Joseph. In the fall of the same
year, Hohenlohe traveled to Rome. On November 27, 1816, the prince was
granted an audience with Pope Pius VII. The Pope began the meeting with
a request to see Hohenlohe's letters of permission, *litterae dismissoriales,*
from the bishop for his leave of absence. Surprised by this turn of events,
the prince excused himself, saying that it was not customary in Germany
to obtain them. The Pope, showing his displeasure with the prince and his
country, tartly replied, "In Germany, there are many things which should
be customary and are not."[16]

Among other things, the Pope was shocked and angry to learn that the prince had administered confession to women at his young age, as church rules at the time forbade priests younger than thirty from hearing confessions by women. The Pope chastised the young prince, but Hohenlohe replied that he had done so only because of the shortage of priests in Germany. This and other practices of which he had been accused would have placed the prince in violation of Catholic doctrine, and the Pope was reserved at first but became more charmed by the young man as the visit progressed. The visit ended on a positive note, and Prince Hohenlohe began his journey home.[17]

On his way, he stopped in Munich where he was invited to preach before King Maximilian Joseph and Crown Prince Ludwig, later to become King Ludwig I. These sermons were very popular with the people; however, trouble arose when the prince's uncle reportedly refused to see him anymore because he accused Hohenlohe of being a pathological liar who told fantasy stories as if they were real. An official report from the nuncio also stated that the prince was forced to leave Munich because he successfully converted to Catholicism the prominent Baron von Schenk and tried to convert the Protestant queen, Frederica Caroline Wilhelmina.

Prince Hohenlohe was also reported to have accumulated a huge debt, which local supporters had to clear for him. Furthermore, a letter from Severoli contained a veiled allegation of an improper relationship with a well-known lady. On June 20, 1817, Hohenlohe was promoted to the clerical council of Bamberg, and he began his duties there in mid-August 1817.[18] Two summers later, in July 1819, the first public controversy involving the prince erupted. Late one night, Hohenlohe was awakened by a summons from the wife of a dying man, Dr. Karl Wetzel, the Protestant editor of the newspaper *Fränkische Merkur.* The charismatic young priest offered such kind spiritual support that the editor agreed to convert to Catholicism. Following a hurried instruction in the basics of the faith, Prince Hohenlohe baptized Dr. Wetzel, heard his confession, and administered the sacraments in the presence of Mrs. Wetzel. Conflicting reports immediately began to circulate, as the editor unexpectedly recovered his strength and then renounced his conversion.

Different contemporary sources commented on the events. The *Weimarer Oppositionsblatte* published an article with a title that roughly translates as, "Hardly believable humbug regarding the conversion of Dr. Wetzel in Bamberg to the Catholic Church." The prince was compelled to defend himself with a document that, in English, is titled, "Forced defense of Prince Alexander von Hohenlohe, curate of the diocese of Bamberg regarding the essay in the *Weimarer Oppositionsblatte* of the year 1819, number 73, titled 'Hardly Believable etc.,'" in which he defended his character and church. Hohenlohe was the subject of intensified scrutiny by local Würzburg authorities, which would ultimately force the prince's departure from Bamberg in the months before the Mattingly cure in Washington.[19]

Meanwhile, the controversial partnership the prince formed with Martin Michel two years later culminated in the dramatic restoration of Mathilde von Schwarzenberg in 1821. The day after she was cured, the general commissioner of the Untermainkreis, Baron Franz Wilhelm von Asbeck, sent a note from Würzburg to the minister of inner affairs in Munich, complaining that the cure of the princess "has attracted a lot of attention" and that Mathilde was now "entirely healthy and fit."[20] Public officials were scrambling to develop an appropriate response to these events.

The county office of Gerlachsheim in Baden, which had been ordered during the police investigation into the cure of Mathilde von Schwarzenberg to issue a witness statement regarding Martin Michel, was not able to report anything to Michel's disadvantage. He was, according to the report, a prosperous, righteous, intelligent farmer with solid knowledge in agrarian issues and a successful vintner. The investigator noted that he had made a good marriage and was a fervent Catholic, free of prejudice and fanatical ideas, but he was a strong believer in the power of exorcism. News of the princess's miraculous cure traveled fast. Soon, crowds of sick people were thronging Prince Hohenlohe, all of them hoping to be healed in a similar way. On June 22, he reportedly cured a paralyzed woman. On June 25, the wife of a blacksmith at the Haug Monastery petitioned him to cure her deafness. The prince told her to kneel down. He then put his hands on her, prayed over her for several minutes, and told her to stand up. At that mo-

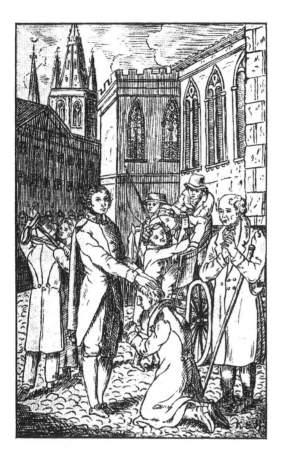

Prince Alexander Hohenlohe healing in the streets of Bamberg (from Hohenlohe's biography by Ludwig Sebastian, 1918).

ment, she shouted that she heard the church clock striking. Word of these additional miracles only added to the excitement surrounding the prince. An early-twentieth-century drawing depicts him in rather dramatic attire, laying hands on an invalid kneeling before him.[21]

In the days following the healing of Princess Mathilde, the excitement about the prince and his humble partner continued to grow. The vicar of Bamberg wrote to Rome on June 26, 1821: "For God's honor, I hope these miracles (*miracoli*) will be accepted as such as it is determined by the holy Canons and as Pope Benedikt XIV has further explained . . . Therefore, I thought it to be my duty to mention my wish to Mr. Fichtl so that the Holy Curate of Würzburg would examine them (miracles) according to the rules of the Holy Council of Trent." The vicar was eager to settle the question of whether the events swirling around Prince Hohenlohe were miracle or mysticism. But the elderly Rev. Fichtl never sent the request, possibly because the orthopedist Dr. Heine never provided the necessary notarized report.[22]

In a series of letters written from Würzburg beginning on June 27, 1821, Francis Nicholas Baur described the commotion surrounding Prince Hohenlohe. According to Baur, the prince gave sermons in the Church of Haug on June 17, before the healing of Princess Mathilde, and three days afterward, on June 24; "many passages of his pious discourses drew abundant tears from the audience," Baur remarked on the prince's magnetic and sympathetic personality that, by his account, drew thousands of people to the town by June 28, and seventy cures were reported. Even the military could not contain the crowds. On June 30, he wrote: "Carriages of all descriptions are continually arriving by all the gates of the city with cripples, lame, blind, and deaf, from distant parts of the Lower Main, as well as from foreign countries, where the influx is increased every day. Some apprehension is entertained for the health of the Prince, on account of his continued exertion." In late June 1821, the prince was performing cures on demand, as many as half a dozen every thirty minutes.[23]

Crown Prince Ludwig himself, who lived in Würzburg at the time, asserted in a letter to Baron von Seinsheim that the prince had entirely cured him of his deafness (see Chapter 2). He wrote:

> Miracles do happen! In the last ten days of last month we in Würzburg thought we had been taken back to the times of the apostles. The deaf can hear—the blind can see—the paralyzed can walk.—Not by having been touched, but by prayer and an invocation in the name of Jesus.—Hohenlohe demands only belief that the supplicant will be helped.—Belief is a mandatory prerequisite. By the evening of the 28th, the number of cured people of all sexes, ages and ranks, was already up to over

seventy, from the lowest to the highest, including myself, the Crown Prince, who had been hard of hearing since childhood. I regained my hearing at noon of the 27th, only a few minutes after the young priest—Prince von Hohenlohe-Schillingsfürst, had said the prayer. I still can't hear as well as others, but it is a vast difference from how well I could hear before; and since then, my ability continues to improve. This young priest is modest and is amazed by his God-given gift. In my waiting room, he cured a woman who had been blind for twenty-five years during his third attempt . . . These are only a few examples of many. My ears are now very sensitive; the sound of the parade last Friday was too loud; for the first time I had to close my windows . . . The people of Würzburg were very enthusiastic about all these events. You can show this letter to every one and have it copied. We live in very interesting times . . . in so many ways.[24]

Prince Hohenlohe was an honored guest at Ludwig's dinner table, where Ludwig remarked, "How happy I am that I can now hear the birds sing and the clock strike." Ludwig provided space in his palace in Würzburg for more healing sessions. The prince was even able to effect cures that Martin Michel had failed to perform, including a woman suffering from gout. A blind woman gave dramatic evidence of being healed when she picked up a cross from the table where she had prayed with her children and shouted: "Look, I can see! Isn't this a lovely cross?" In another stunning episode, the prince healed a student who had to be carried about in a wagon, and the young man was able to rise up and walk. The same day, Baron Franz Wilhelm von Asbeck reported to the Ministry of Affairs, "Dealing with the events, as they have presented themselves over the past few days, is of a delicate nature that demands calmness and careful actions . . . especially, since it is quite true that many deaf people can now hear, many blind people can now see and many people with gout are now free of all pain." Von Asbeck also reported on the prince's powerful sermons that were attracting more followers, so many that the prince himself requested police protection.[25]

But Prince Hohenlohe was not successful at every healing attempt. One afternoon, he tried to heal eighteen sick people at Würzburg's Julius Hospital in front of a group of doctors. Johann Georg Heine was in attendance, and none of the patients improved. The director gleefully noted that there was not even the slightest change in any of them. Heine must have felt vindicated, given his previous attempt to deflect credit away from the prince in the cure of Mathilde von Schwarzenberg.[26]

Prince Hohenlohe left Würzburg on July 1, 1821, and arrived in Bamberg the next day. On his way, several vehicles full of sick people were heading in the direction of Würzburg, and he reportedly got out of his carriage and healed them. The number of people seeking help from him grew so large that police needed to control the crowds in local towns whenever he passed through them. In Bamberg, especially, numerous sick people thronged the town. On July 5, a police officer wrote to the commanding officer in Bayreuth:

> Curate Prince von Hohenlohe arrived from Würzburg on July 2, and on the following day performed several cures in private homes of different sick people by praying for them and reminding them to renew the strength of their belief in God. These included people who had suffered from gout for eight or nine years and had not left their beds during that time. Once the prayer was finished, they were able to get up and walk immediately. Because this drew attention, people, not only from the city but also from the surrounding countryside, some from as far away as six or seven hours, gathered at the place where Hohenlohe was staying. There he cured several more: he made the blind see, the deaf hear, and the lame walk. These extraordinary circumstances caused a crowd of several thousand people to gather, and the curate was no longer able to perform the healings in his own room. He went outside on the commons to perform his deeds.

Like some town officials, the police were themselves uncertain how best to proceed in this unusual circumstance. While the officials in Würzburg had acted rather hesitantly, the magistrate of the city of Bamberg, especially the mayor, Franz Ludwig von Hornthal, was not willing to patiently witness the commotion without acting on it. An increasingly contentious atmosphere developed between the prince and the mayor, the son of a Jewish rabbi who had converted to Catholicism. He wryly observed, "Our police laws are not designed to react to a case as strange as this one."[27]

After another short visit in Würzburg, the now famous Hohenlohe arrived in the mountain spa of Bad Brückenau on July 12 and visited Crown Prince Ludwig. A member of the gendarmerie of Brückenau described the attempts to cure that took place on July 15: "Today, Sunday, a large crowd of people, many had come from far off places, and gathered on the plaza. There were several thousand people and up to eighty-nine carriages and fifty-seven horses were counted; several of that crowd had been cured by the prince, the guest of our dear crown prince, in public through prayer and the touch of his hand." One commentator observed, "A sorrowful picture of human suffering was witnessed by the citizens of the town." The cured included Catholics, Protestants, and Jews. A little chapel in Schillings-fürst still has a collection of crutches and a placard that reads, "crutches of those who, immediately after calling Jesus's name, with the help of Prince Alexander von Hohenlohe, Schillingsfürst, were cured in the summer of 1821."[28]

Mindful of the Vatican's response to his healings, Prince Hohenlohe wrote to Pope Pius VII for advice on how to use his gift and asked the church to take a position on the miracles. The prince was not the only one who was eager to hear what the Pope thought. On July 26, the apostolic vicar wrote to Rome: "The Lord shall be delighted that Hohenlohe's cures honor Him and happen for the good of the church. But still, one needs to fear the opposite. He knows neither good measure nor tact when he attempts them. He thinks himself able to cure sick people by the dozen any hour, day and night. Up to now he has ignored my good advice, and has ignored the degrees of the government to organize his attempts to cure. The entire community of clergy fears the worst of effects for our church and our religion as a result of such inconsiderate activity. I dearly await the decision of our

Holy See on this matter." The Holy See's position on the miracles would largely determine how they would be received.[29]

The healings caused extraordinary excitement and created polarization among the prince's contemporaries. For his critics, his cures signaled a relapse into irrationality and religious fanaticism; for believers, the cures were signs of God's mercy and demonstrative love. The restorations involved the highest authorities of the church (Pius VII) and the state (King Maximilian Joseph I) in a challenging situation trying to manage Prince Hohenlohe and his doings. One public official, Constantin Ludwig von Welden, worried that "during a time in which dangerous inclinations of a religious nature have threatened peace among the states, this newly fashionably religious romanticism has the dangerous potential of causing new religious conflicts." The controversies surrounding the prince threatened a delicate balance. Strict regulations on his activities were put into place by civil authorities: first, the patient's priest must be in the room; second, the circumstances of the disease and the personal data of the sick person must be reviewed; and third, Hohenlohe's behavior during the curing attempts must be reported to government officials. The prince promised the president of the vicariate to obey the guidelines, but he frequently did not.[30]

One of Hohenlohe's biographers, C. G. Scharold, wrote a series of letters from Würzburg during August 1821 that detail many of the dramatic incidents that followed the healing of Princess Mathilde von Schwarzenberg. He reported that crowds from as far away as Franconia and Swabia were hurrying to see Prince Hohenlohe in Bad Brückenau in northern Bavaria. The spa's sour-tasting well water had been famous for at least four centuries for its curative powers, and the town had become a favorite retreat of Crown Prince Ludwig of Bavaria, who had overseen several renovations to the resort. Scharold reported seeing a sign posted near the tavern of Oberleichtersbach, located on a country road approximately one hour from the spa that warned:

> By order of the kingship of the Lower Main River District, all
> local officials are instructed to inform all citizens and foreigners

who wish to be healed by Prince von Hohenlohe that they will not be allowed to travel into the spa. Moreover, citizens must carry proof in the form of a medical certificate describing their illness and foreigners have to carry a passport or other official document to prove their identity, otherwise they will be turned away. Officials are furthermore instructed to transmit this information not only to the community but also to all churches and parish halls that they be required to post it. —Brückenau, July 22, 1821. The Royal Provincial Court.[31]

Local officials were tightening a net of regulations around the prince.

Scharold arrived on July 28 and found the little chapel where Prince Hohenlohe was saying Mass. It was overflowing with invalids hoping for a cure. When the Mass ended, the aspirants refused to leave the church, pleading with the prince to take pity on them. He spoke to them saying: "Who allowed you to come here? Do you not know that this is prohibited? I must follow my orders and obey my instructions. I cannot expose myself to punishment." The clamorous pleading of the sick only increased, so the prince, touched by compassion, started listening. He took off his priestly garments and stood on the steps of the altar, sweating profusely. He began with his typical brief admonition about faith and trust, and then he bent forward in devotion to all the hundreds seeking help. According to Scharold, the prince met with them, one by one. He noted that those sick with gout were healed easily and quickly. Deaf and blind people demanded longer and repeated prayers, and other, more serious ailments required the most time. Those who were successfully cured were instructed by the prince to remain in the chapel and to thank God for the favor. He advised those who could not be helped, or who had been helped only slightly, to have more faith and grow in goodness in order to receive help if it was God's will and their fate. Many left the little chapel comforted and calmed, Scharold wrote, with tears of joy in their eyes.[32]

The prince had been in Brückenau for about ten days, and the prohibitions against his healing had been issued. But the crowds kept coming, hordes and hordes of sick people descending on the little town. There were days, according to Scharold, when thousands of people gathered underneath the trees of the marketplace and begged the prince for help. Military forces were called in to try to restore order. The streets were so filled with sick people that mail could not be delivered to the town. Crowds continued to throng around the prince, and there were many more alleged healings of Catholics, Lutherans, and Reformists. The prince made a side trip to the nearby town of Fulda, where more healings were attributed to him. On August 9, he left Bad Brückenau to return to Bamberg. On the way, he was welcomed to Würzburg by a song composed by university students, who presented him with a wreath of flowers. During his three-day stay in Würzburg, several more remarkable healings were reported.[33]

When Prince Hohenlohe returned to Bamberg on August 13, 1821, Mayor von Hornthal was dismayed that the commotion had not subsided. On September 7, the Bavarian Council of Ministers ordered the newspapers not to report on Hohenlohe's doings. They hoped that silencing the press might cause the frenzy over his miracle working to fade. The controversy surrounding Hohenlohe eventually became so heated that the king of Bavaria contacted the nuncio Francesco Serra-Cassano in September, requesting that Hohenlohe be recalled to Rome until the excitement in Bavaria had calmed.

When the long-awaited letter from the Pope arrived on September 8, it was not very definitive: "We admire the healings of our beloved Son, the Clerical Council Prince Alexander von Hohenlohe, and encourage him to continue those without causing a sensation so that the holiness will not become a subject of curiosity and mockery." These words foreshadow the same concerns that Archbishop Maréchal would express following the Mattingly miracle of 1824. The Pope, at this moment, saw no reason to prohibit prayers for the sick; however, he ordered the prince to avoid generating any more publicity that might draw ridicule to holy rituals. The letter continued: "We expect an accurate and faithful collection of the most important healings accompanied by an affidavit of confirmation. Thereupon, we will call a special committee that will decide about the miraculous nature of those healings after a thorough investigation is performed. Until further notice we give our beloved son the apostolic blessing."[34]

This letter suggests that the Vatican was willing to begin its complex process of documentation to certify the veracity of the miracles of Prince Alexander Hohenlohe. For more than four hundred years, the Roman Catholic Church has probed miracles attributed to prospective saints through the careful collection of evidence. Inquiries into miraculous healings consist of a rigorous "trial" that involves the assembling of forensic evidence that a miracle has occurred. Since the Tridentine reforms of 1588, the canonization process has scrutinized two main aspects of such events: the first, a close examination of the supposedly exemplary life of the candidate for sainthood, and the second, proof that the would-be saint worked miracles. Hohenlohe's contemporaries were willing to begin this process in 1821, as Bishop John England would also do in the United States a decade later with his investigation of the Mattingly miracle.[35]

The prince was encouraged by the Pope's support and read the letter with tears of gratitude. That day, Scharold reported, Hohenlohe cured a highly ranked official of the Austrian Treasury. The treasurer had been suffering from a dislocation of the left hip for ten years, caused by a twelve-foot fall. His leg had been so weak from the hip down that it had to be supported by a bandage, and he walked, in constant pain, with both a crutch and a cane. After the prince said a short prayer over him, the treasurer returned to his guesthouse, threw away the crutch, the cane, and the bandage, and walked around freely and painlessly. The old and invigorated Hungarian returned to his rescuer with tears of joy and gratitude rolling down his cheeks, where they fell and wet the prince's consecrating hand that he was reverently kissing.[36]

The local authorities clashed with national and church authorities when Emperor Franz I of Austria demanded that all bishops and curators open all cathedrals to allow Hohenlohe, should he come to their dioceses, to perform his cures in the cathedrals. The emperor, whose daughter Marie Louise had married Napoleon in 1810, also ordered the police to give the miracle worker all the support he needed. Word of the prince's healings soon spread to France in the journal *L'Ami de la Religion et du Roi,* and then to Hungary, Bohemia, Poland, and Prussia. Letters from the sick in these regions began to flood the mail, and the prince responded by promising to pray for them at specific times. Several cures were reported by those who followed the prince's instructions: a medical doctor of twenty-five years' experience whose eye ailment was cured, the ten-year-old daughter of a customs official who recovered her ability to walk, and a woman whose lameness was cured.

Material in the Vatican archives shows that Rome issued a secret directive on August 25, 1821, in which it advised the nuncio Serra-Cassano to obtain, either himself or with the help of others, deeper knowledge of Hohenlohe's way of life, his habits, and his beliefs, mainly his religious ideals, so that any suspicions could be eradicated. The nuncio was to proceed in the same manner regarding Hohenlohe's helper named "M.M." (Martin Michel), whom the vicar of Bamberg had called a "frequent visitor" of the taverns. He was also asked to gather detailed information on some of the cures that had received a lot of attention, especially those that had at first been called "miracle" but then had been refuted. Finally, he was to collect the various opinions of the most intelligent and reputable Catholics on these cures. When everything was collected in this matter, he would be able to compose a final report that could be given to the Pope so that he could examine the matter and reach a final decision on how to deal with this supposed miracle worker. Thus, the detailed process of verifying miracles according to Tridentine rules had begun.[37]

In late August, Crown Prince Ludwig, whose deafness reportedly had been cured by Prince Hohenlohe, argued with his father King Maximilian over the prince. Tensions flared when Prince Hohenlohe wrote to the king asking for a restoration of a stipend of 1,800 gulden that the king had formerly provided for him until he became curate of Bamberg. This request so angered Maximilian that he rebuked the prince and said he would give the money to the needy instead. The king also ordered that no mention of Prince Hohenlohe be made before him, which essentially banned news of the prince's doings from court.[38]

On September 4, an official announcement appeared in the newspaper *Allgemeine Zeitung* signed by von Hornthal, City Magistrate, who had called Hohenlohe's cures *Afterwunderkram* (asinine miracle stuff): "We order these attempts to stop so that we can prevent deceit as well as accumulations of large crowds of sick people, beggars, cripples and wanderers and others. Our orders have the approval of the highest authorities. We have advised P. v. H. to scrupulously obey these orders." Von Hornthal then restated some of the strictures imposed on the prince. Furthermore, von Hornthal stated: "We publicly announce this decision so that people traveling here from afar will not lose time and money endangering themselves by embarking on this journey. We will not allow any attempts to cure by the prince under these circumstances, and have threatened him with punishment if he disobeys this order. We add, that all earlier attempts made by P. v. H. that were made in the presence of the commission or of one or more physicians were unsuccessful. Those attempts called miracles only took place in the absence of any supervision, without the knowledge of the sick people or the diseases, in secret or in very public and crowded places." Despite von Hornthal's efforts, near riots broke out in early September. Another newspaper, *Neckar Zeitung,* followed up with this comment: "Bamberg, Sept. 12th: The miracle factory of P. v. H. is now without work. His products were very popular in the beginning, but now the customers have left." A week later, the same newspaper published a claim that one of the cured was back in his wheelchair, but a published letter from a high Munich official disputed that claim.[39]

Throughout the excitement, the prince maintained that he would abide by the wishes of the Pope in regards to the cures. He was, however, unable to avoid drawing attention to himself despite the clear admonition from the Vatican. Prince Hohenlohe declined to receive a letter from von Hornthal stating restrictions on his actions, saying that he could not accept delivery as his title was missing from the address. Von Hornthal replied in an angry letter to the Ministry of Inner Affairs that the prince had a tendency to force his "so-called miracles" on people and "threaten the enlightened German state with the creation of darkness." In another statement he wrote, "We think the disease of Prince Hohenlohe is contagious, and if not treated it can be detrimental to public order." Prince Hohenlohe complained to the king that these restrictions were offensive. The angry king had a copy made of the prince's letter and then tore it to pieces and returned it to the prince.[40]

Finally, under pressure from civil authorities, the prince decided to cease his attempts to cure and addressed the Bavarian public in the newspaper *Fränkische Merkur* on October 14, 1821. In an open letter to all clergy, he requested that they not send any more sick people to him, citing the demands of his own parish work and his delicate health. During this period, however, Hohenlohe intensified the contacts he maintained via the mail with people from several foreign countries who requested his help. In response, he would write a few lines recommending that the sick have boundless confidence that their prayers would be heard. On preprinted stationery, he appointed a time that he would unite in prayer with the sick. He also recommended a novena in honor of the holy name of Jesus. It was one of these letters that eventually found its way to Washington, D.C., and into the hands of Ann Mattingly's friends.[41]

Hohenlohe, however, did not completely discontinue his healing work. On February 18, 1822, the magistrate of the city of Bamberg reported to the government of the Obermainkreis: "That he, to this day, and especially after he moved into his apartment, continues to attempt cures in secret is known to us, but since he was staying out of the public's eye, we saw no need to act against him; for some time now, the publicity, especially the pamphlet created by vicar Baur of Würzburg about Hohenlohe's miraculous cures, which is now translated into Dutch, is circulating and attracting supplicants from different towns; even from different countries. People are pouring in to visit him. Of course, those who have not been helped have to return home without hope and at great expense. Not only foreigners, but also those unhappy ones who live close by gather around him." Prince Hohenlohe's confrontations with Mayor von Hornthal grew more heated as a circuslike atmosphere prevailed in the town, despite the civil restrictions and the prince's own expressed wishes.[42]

On May 22, 1822, Hohenlohe petitioned the king and the archbishop of Bamberg, Baron von Stubenberg, for a three-month leave to visit his mother in Vienna. He arrived there on May 30, with hordes of sick people following him. At Passau, in southeast Germany, thousands thronged the bridge over the Danube to escort the prince to church, where it was reported he remained blessing the sufferers until 2 A.M. He went on to extend his stay in the city of the emperor without asking for further permission. On September 21, the prince had an audience with Tsar Alexander I of Russia in Vienna. The prince and tsar agreed to keep the long, confidential conversation secret, but reportedly, the tsar fell on his knees before Prince Hohenlohe to receive his blessing.[43]

In 1822, the prince forged another association that would be of great assistance to him. Reverend Joseph Forster (1790–1875) became a devotee of his when Hohenlohe cured a relative of Forster's of a throat disease. Forster was the pastor of Huttenheim, and Prince Hohenlohe installed himself at the rectory there and entrusted Forster with his confidence and correspondence. But Forster was unprepared for the challenges that followed in the wake of his association with Prince Hohenlohe, as his little office was flooded with letters from foreign countries requesting the prayers of the prince. At first, he tried to answer them individually, but the torrent of mail became so great that it was soon impossible for him to read them all. To respond efficiently, Forster began sending notices to various districts and foreign countries, announcing days that Prince Hohenlohe would remember the sick who wished to join him in prayer. Biographer Ludwig Sebastian reported seeing a Hohenlohe collection at the Royal Library and the Historical Club in Bamberg that held several prayer notes. One had the prince's instructions to Forster on the back: "All French on July 25th at 8 o'clock, all Germans on July 26th at 8 o'clock. Also, please sign with my name."[44]

But still, there were the crowds of sick to contend with. The sheer numbers of suffering people descending on the town of Huttenheim made Forster compare his rectory to an open dovecote. In desperation, he pinned a note to the rectory door that stated, "All visitors who are not concerned with parish or official business will not be admitted." He harshly chastised any who ignored the sign, but nothing stopped the petitioners. At times, when the prince was traveling and supplicants besieged Forster, he would try to cure them himself.[45]

In the Eyes of His Contemporaries

The controversy over the cures in Germany mirrored some of the themes of the controversy in the United States. Some German Catholics believed that in a time of declining religious belief, miracles were necessary to glorify the church. Dr. Friedrich Brenner of Bamberg, a Catholic theologian, pointed out that those criteria that the Catholic Church had established in order to determine miracles had not been met in Hohenlohe's attempts to cure people. True miraculous powers, he said, are limited by nothing, whereas Hohenlohe, as he himself admitted, could not cure all diseases. The prince's prayer cures often proved to be only partly successful, or the disease returned after a short period. God does not perform miracles for the moment, Brenner maintained, and Hohenlohe's cures had to be seen as natural effects.[46]

The prince's former professor, Peter Aloys Gratz, of Ellwangen, went further, writing that "the facts had not always been correctly determined. Those who believed in the 'miracle' had only reported on successful cures, even the type of disease was not always known." The professor attributed some of the cures to the patients' willpower. Like Brenner, another critic, Gratz also asserted that the prince carefully chose the types of disease he would attempt to cure, suggesting that the healings depended on psychological effects. Gratz regarded Prince Hohenlohe as a zealot in whom, through the transparent coat of humility, a holy pride could be seen. As would be the case in Washington, D.C., some worried that these actions caused controversy that every reasonable Catholic should deplore. Furthermore, contemporary German Protestant theologians nearly always concluded that the prince had not performed any miracles at all.[47]

And there were the criticisms of the prince's behavior in his personal life. Paul Johann von Feuerbach, an official at the Appeals Court in Ansbach, wrote to Elise von der Recke in August 1821 that Prince Hohenlohe "is in his relations to the other gender a deeply dissipated man, who seduces girls, attempts to abort children, and is not shy about bragging of his dissipation in certain circles. Duke L told me himself that at his dinner table Hohenlohe revealed how on his way to Rome (forgive me the inappropriateness for the truth's sake) he lost his virginity. Now he lives in Bamberg with an overly pious pretty woman in highly familiar circumstances." Ludwig Sebastian, the prince's biographer, concluded that these strong accusations were unjustified, but lingering doubts about the prince's behavior made him an unlikely candidate for Catholic sainthood, and his name was never further advanced.[48]

Westward over the Ocean

During 1822 and 1823, news of Prince Hohenlohe's miraculous cures was wending its way westward. Word of mouth and Rev. Forster's letters had reached France, England, and Ireland, where a number of cures were reported. In France, twelve people witnessed one of the prince's cures at the Convent of St. Benoit in Toulouse. A nun named Adelaide Veysre had suffered for six months after an injury to her leg had twisted her foot nearly around. She asked the cardinal bishop of Toulouse to apply to Prince Hohenlohe for help, and he wrote the prince in May 1822. The prince replied that on July 25, the feast of St. James, he would pray for Veysre's recovery. At the same time, the bishop performed Mass in the nun's room, and, it was claimed, when he raised the Host, her foot resumed its proper position. Eventually, she recovered completely.[49]

The prince's fame spread to England, and on January 3, 1822, this advertisement appeared in the newspapers:

> To Germans, Foreign Merchants, and Others.—Prince Alexander of Hohenlohe.—Whereas several public journals, both foreign and domestic, have announced most extraordinary cures to have been performed by Prince Alexander of Hohenlohe: This is to entreat that any one who can give unerring information

concerning him, where he now is, or of his intended route, will immediately do so: and they will thereby confer on a female, labouring under what is considered an incurable malady, an obligation which no words can describe. Should a gentleman give the information, his own feelings would sufficiently recompense him: but if a person in indigent circumstances, ten guineas will with pleasure be given, provided the correctness of his information can be ascertained.—Address to A. B., at Mrs. Hedge's, Laundress, 9, Mount Row, Davies Street, Berkeley Square.[50]

Rich and poor, then, sought out the favors of Prince Hohenlohe, and their desperation is poignant.

One of the first cures to take place in England, on May 3, 1822, was that of Barbara O'Connor, an Irish-born nun in a convent in Chelmsford, Essex, who was in her early thirties. For several years, O'Connor had been affected with swelling in her hand and arm that worsened over time. Several doctors were unsuccessful in curing the condition in which her "fingers looked ready to burst, and the wrist fifteen inches in circumference." At length, the convent's superior, having heard of Prince Hohenlohe's powers, wrote to him, soliciting his prayers and advice. The prince replied that on May 3, at eight o'clock in the morning, O'Connor should make confession, take Communion, and offer up her own fervent prayers; the prince promised to pray for her at the same time. O'Connor did as directed, and her pains left her. According to O'Connor's testimony, she heard a sudden crack in her right shoulder, from which a thrilling sensation darted to the ends of her fingers. The pain ceased, and she recovered the use of her arm and hand. Her doctors were unable to offer a medical explanation. This occurred just two years before Mrs. Mattingly's cure on the other side of the Atlantic.[51]

During the summer and autumn of 1823, a number of additional cures took place in Ireland. News of Barbara O'Connor's cure had spread and attracted the attention of James Lalor, whose eighteen-year-old daughter Maria had not spoken in six years following what he called a "severe and protracted illness." He solicited the help of Rev. James Warren Doyle,

Bishop of Kildare, who wrote to Prince Hohenlohe about the case. Maria Lalor, the bishop told the prince, was a pious young woman who deserved God's help. She followed Hohenlohe's standard instructions: repent and confess beforehand, be confident of a recovery, receive Communion, and resolve to lead an exemplary life afterward. As in the Washington case to come, attempts were made to time the Mass that followed the nine days of prayer with Prince Hohenlohe's service in Bamberg. Maria Lalor received Communion on June 11, 1823; then she reported hearing a voice that said, "Mary, you are well." She exclaimed, "O Lord! Am I?" and threw herself face down in adoration. She was afterwards able to speak in a clear and distinct voice.[52]

A few weeks later, Mary Stuart, a Carmelite nun in St. Joseph's Convent, Ranelagh, was cured of attacks of paralysis that had plagued her for four and a half years, leaving her bedridden and unable to speak. Two priests and four nuns joined her in Mass, and on August 1, she was healed through the intersession of Prince Hohenlohe. The prince designated Monday, September 1, 1823, as the day he would single out the sick of Ireland. Crowds flocked to local churches, and there were several reports of cures: a blind man in Kildare suddenly could see; Mary Scully, also of County Kildare, was cured of ten years of ulcers and pain; James Kelly, age twenty-six, was cured after six years of illness that his doctors had determined was incurable; Miss Dowell from Dublin was restored from a host of unspecified infirmities; and the shoemaker Michael Read, also of Dublin, recovered from a rheumatic affliction.[53]

Daniel O'Connell, the rising political and legal star, became a believer and took the Dublin miracles as a sign that God was favoring Irish Catholics. O'Connell is remembered in Ireland as the founder of the Catholic Association, which campaigned for emancipation and mobilized the Catholic community, with the help of the clergy, to become a political force. O'Connell was a particularly strong advocate for supernatural agency. The miracles during the summer of 1823 in Ireland were highly politicized, with O'Connell claiming that they proved that God was on the side of Catholics. These healings, and two pastoral letters that trumpeted them by James War-

ren Doyle, bishop of Kildare and Leighlin, and Daniel Murray, archbishop
of Dublin, began to be viewed by Irish Protestants as instruments of Catholic subversion. According to historian Laurence M. Geary, the controversial
prophecies of the English Benedictine Charles Walmesley (1722–1797), who
used the pseudonym Signor Pastorini to predict an apocalyptic end to Protestant rule in Ireland, were wrapped up in the strong antipathy to Doyle's
pastoral letter about the Hohenlohe miracles. An editorial in the Protestant
Warder warned, "Prophecies and miracles, priests and demagogues, the
schools of the Jesuits, and the harangues of the Catholic Association, are
all in full co-operation, ripening and fructifying to a harvest of civil dissention, of anarchy and blood." The controversy swirling around the cures
of Prince Hohenlohe in Ireland were in some ways a foreshadowing of the
debates surrounding the cure of Ann Mattingly in 1824. The question of
whose side God favored, the Catholics or the Protestants, took on resonance
in the United States as it had in Ireland.[54]

An Orange newspaper adapted the popular ballad "Green Grow the
Rushes O" to the following words:

> Now let all pious Christians pray
> For these deluded people O
> Who humbug lasses, with their masses,
> In church without a steeple O
> May crucifix and bag of tricks,
> And darkness vanish from our land,
> And in their place, may faith, with grace
> Stop miracles and sleight of hand.[55]

As the mention of "lasses" in this parody demonstrates, the events took on
some of the typical gendered interpretations of the day, claiming that hys-
terical women were especially susceptible to superstitious machinations.

It is likely that news of the miracles passed first among various religious communities and then in the international press. Through these
channels, word of the prince's wonderworking reached the United States.

Fewer than six months before the cure of Ann Mattingly, a newspaper in Schenectady, New York, published a satirical commentary called "Lord Norbery and the Irish Miracle." At the opening of the Queen's County assizes, Lord Norbery, in charging the grand jury, alluded to the recent miracle of Prince Hohenlohe that restored Maria Lalor's ability to speak. "'If,' said his lordship, 'a female has been brought to the recovery of her speech in this county, God be praised; but as great a miracle has been performed in another county, (Carlow,) where Moll Doyle has been made perfectly silent.' (Shouts of laughter.) He was glad to see even the humblest men in the community laugh when he talked of the 'miracle.'" In addition to demonstrating how widespread knowledge of the prince was even six months before the Mattingly miracle, this anecdote underlines again the significance of gender in the miracle cures.[56]

But in France, England, Ireland, and the United States, the faithful did not know that the wonder worker himself was under siege. In June 1822, after the prince had left Bamberg, the Pope sent a request to the Bavarian bishops to investigate whether or not miraculous cures of substance had occurred in other dioceses. In the archdiocese of Bamberg, 124 dioceses reported mostly unsuccessful cures. Twenty-two dioceses reported having no one who had undergone an attempt. These were apparently the final results; the Vatican never concluded an investigation. It is not clear why none of the alleged *miraculées,* or cured, stepped forward. Perhaps they or their clergy were encouraged to make the results inconclusive. Prince Hohenlohe's behavior had put him at odds with both church and local officials, and letting the controversy die out likely seemed the prudent course.[57]

In December 1822, the ordinariat of Bamberg voiced his dismay over the prince's unauthorized long absence from his parish and requested that he return to his post. Prince Hohenlohe replied one month later, saying he had received a confirmation of a position in Hungary and therefore gave up his position in Bamberg. By January 1823, then, he had fully relinquished his position in the city. He did not take up his next post as head of the cathedral in Grosswardein until April 14, 1825, more than a year after his purported cure of Ann Mattingly. During the time that the group in Washington was carefully timing their novenas and Masses with the prince's schedule, he was actually on an extended vacation, in between clerical appointments. Ironically, the Washington group had postponed attempting the cure in February because the prince's letter had arrived after the date of the Mass on the tenth. Though Archbishop Maréchal feared it might well be the case, it would be a long time before anyone was able to confirm that Prince Hohenlohe was not in Bamberg on March 10, 1824, offering Mass for the sick in North America.

FIVE

A Capital Miracle

Against those miracle-mongers, my God hath put me on my guard,
by admonishing me that in the last days there shall arise *false prophets*,
who shall work such signs and wonders as to deceive, if possible, the very elect.

—St. Augustine, quoted in *The Christian Observer* (1818)

Western Virginia, 1797

One night, when clouds scudded over the face of the half moon ahead of a gathering storm, a weary traveler knocked at Adam Livingston's door, in Smithfield, in the western part of Virginia. Livingston lived with his wife, three sons, and four daughters on a seventy-acre farm half a mile west of Smithfield, today known as Middleway. The town stood at the crossroads of several highways, and it was not unusual for strangers who could not secure a room at the busy village inn to seek shelter at the Livingston farm as they headed westward. The Livingstons gave the man a meal and a room, and the pale stranger retired to his bed. During the night, loud wheezing and coughing coming from the stranger's room awakened the family. The man had become seriously ill. He told Mr. Livingston that he was a Catholic and, fearing he may be dying, requested that his host call a priest. Livingston, himself a Pennsylvanian-born Lutheran, hated Catholics and told the stranger that he knew of no priest in the neighborhood. He then cruelly remarked to the sick man, "Even if there was one, he should never pass the threshold of my door!"

The stranger's condition deteriorated rapidly, and he continued to cry out for a priest. Livingston did his best to provide what comfort he could to the desperate man in his final moments. After the stranger died, Livingston employed one of his farmhands to sit up with the corpse. The workman lighted candles in the chamber to begin his vigil, but their light quickly dimmed, flickered, and went out, leaving the room in darkness. The man relit them, but again the candles went out, and he concluded that they must be defective. He called Livingston, who brought two tapers that he had been using in his own family room. These were burned down a third of the way already, and he knew them to be good. But as soon as they were lighted in the room with the corpse, they also went out. This so alarmed the farmhand that he abandoned his post and hurried out of the house. The next morning, some neighbors helped Livingston bury the stranger's body in a distant corner of his property. They erected a small cross to mark his grave. From that moment, increasingly strange things began to happen in the home of Adam Livingston.

As the family sat before the fire on the evening of the burial, coals began popping out of the fireplace. Livingston quickly smothered them before they could cause a fire. The next night, as the family sat at dinner, dishes flew out of the cupboards and smashed on the floor. For the next several nights, a sound of galloping horses disturbed the family's sleep, but no horses could be seen anywhere on the property. A week after the stranger's death, Livingston's barn burned to the ground, killing all his cattle. A few weeks after that, an angry teamster stopped his wagon on the road in front of Livingston's house because of ropes blocking the way. Livingston came out to assist, but when the teamster slashed at the cords with his knife, it passed right through them, and the lines appeared to remain taut. In the coming months, Livingston had to persuade passing wagons to ride straight through the ghostly cords that seemed to obstruct the road in front of his property. Some sources say that in the barnyard, the heads simply dropped off Livingston's turkeys and chickens. And a large satchel of money belonging to the family inexplicably vanished from their home.

But none of these strange occurrences compared to the maddening metallic sound that gave the Livingston phenomenon its name: the Wizard Clip. Livingston's house became filled with a whirring noise of scissors snipping. Blankets, boots, clothes, and curtains were cut to tatters. According to local lore, an old Presbyterian woman from nearby Martinsburg came into the house to inspect the Wizard Clip, carefully wrapping her new black silk cap in her handkerchief before entering. When she later unfolded the handkerchief, which was intact, she discovered that her silk cap had been cut to ribbons. Other visitors found that invisible scissors had cut shapes of half-moons and other curiously wrought figures into their clothes. One night, three adventurous young men from a nearby town came to Smithfield, scoffing at the reports they had heard and bragging of their bravery. They offered to sleep in the house all night and to face the devil himself, if he were the author of these doings. As they sat boasting in the main room of the house, a large stone detached itself from the fireplace and whirled around the floor in front of them like a tornado. The three worthies, shrieking in terror, fled back to the safety of their village.

Now on the verge of mental and physical collapse, Adam Livingston went to his minister pleading for help, but the Lutheran clergyman was powerless to stop the supernatural assaults. Several other ministers also made attempts, to no avail, and one unfortunate Methodist had a crock of sour milk poured over his head. Shortly after this, Adam Livingston had a dream. In it, he was struggling to climb a high mountain. He grabbed at roots and bushes and pulled himself upward with enormous effort. At the summit, he saw a beautiful church and an imposing personage before him, "dressed in robes," as he described it. He gazed at the figure and then heard a voice, saying, "This is the man who can relieve you." Lying in the bed beside her husband, Mrs. Livingston heard his groans in his sleep and shook him awake. He told her of his dream, saying that in the morning he would begin searching for the man in robes.

Livingston heard that a Catholic priest would be saying Mass in nearby Shepherdstown the following Sunday and, overcoming his former antipathy, decided to seek him out. On Sunday morning, he waited in a pew in the back of the church. When Rev. Dennis Cahill appeared at the altar, dressed in his vestments, Livingston was nearly overcome. He began to weep and exclaimed: "This is the very man I saw in my dream! He is the one that the voice told me would relieve me from my troubles." When the Mass was over, Livingston promptly called on the priest and told him of the events occurring during the past few years on his farm. At first, Cahill

laughed with disbelief and told Livingston that his neighbors must be playing tricks on him. But then, taking pity on the distraught man, Cahill agreed
to visit Livingston's house and investigate the strange circumstances he had
described. As the priest began looking into the matter, the spooky happenings were corroborated not only by the Livingston family, but also by the
townspeople of Smithfield.

Cahill entered the Livingston house, prayed, and sprinkled it with
holy water. As he turned to leave, the family's missing satchel of money
appeared to drop out of nowhere and fell onto the front step. For a few
days after Cahill's visit, all was quiet, but then the haunting began anew.
By now, the story had spread to the diocese of Baltimore, and Bishop John
Carroll sent Rev. Dmitri Gallitzin to investigate. Gallitzin (1770–1840) was
an émigré Russian prince and Catholic priest today known as the Apostle
of the Alleghenies. Since 2005, he has been under consideration for possible
canonization by the Catholic Church in recognition of the large number of
converts he attracted to the fledgling church. Gallitzin was one of the first
Roman Catholic priests ordained in America in March 1795. He had been
assigned to work in church missions in Maryland. Though Gallitzin sometimes clashed with Bishop Carroll over procedural matters, he ultimately
built up a large congregation in Maryland and Pennsylvania. Born in The
Hague, in Holland, he was the only son of one of the oldest, wealthiest, and
most illustrious families of Russia. Gallitzin's decision to become a Roman
Catholic priest had cost him a rich inheritance, and he served out his life
as a poor parish priest in humble American missions.

Gallitzin moved in with the Livingston family for three months to
investigate the possession of the house by demons. The Russian nobleman
became convinced that Satan needed to be expelled from the house. Doubting his own strength to complete such an undertaking on his own, Gallitzin
joined forces with Cahill, whom he called a "man of powerful nerve and
hearty faith," to perform the ritual of expulsion. Bidding the members of
the household to kneel down, they commanded the evil spirits to leave
the house without doing injury to anyone there. Reportedly, as the devils
resisted, pots and pans and household furnishings flew around the room

to the deafening sound of the whirring scissors, but then fell harmlessly to the floor, conquered by the combined strength of the holy men. Cahill afterward said Mass at the home, and there was no more trouble. For many years, Cahill kept samples of the tattered clothing in a trunk as evidence of the demonic possession.

Adam Livingston and his family converted to Catholicism, and the destructive events in their home subsided, but for the next seventeen years, a mysterious voice could be heard giving instructions in prayer, especially when a death was about to occur. Some say that the Catholic man who died without a priest's blessing was finally appeased. Eventually, Adam Livingston bequeathed his land to the Catholic Church, which still owns it today. Prince Gallitzin's account of his stay with the Livingstons has now been lost, but the legend has been passed down through other sources, including letters written by Annella McSherry, wife of Richard McSherry, who were eyewitnesses to the events at the Livingston farm. In a strange historical coincidence, Ann Mattingly's niece, Helen Mary, daughter of her brother James, married into the McSherry family. The European nobleman, Prince Gallitzin, had worked in concert with the Reverend Cahill, a humble parish priest, to perform an exorcism on the frontier of the new nation. But another European nobleman and priest, Alexander Hohenlohe, would become much more well known for the dramatic event in the nation's capital.[1]

The Cultural Context

Ann Mattingly's miraculous cure was a dynamic event that came to fruition in the early American republic, but its roots in Catholic Europe nourished it. Nearly half a century after the United States had officially severed its ties with England, the European continent still remained a looming presence in the American consciousness, and the Monroe Doctrine of 1823 was a fresh articulation of the continued desire for separation from that continent. European martyrologies and stories that detailed physically graphic suffering by Catholic saints provided a significant context for the documents that were generated after Mrs. Mattingly's healing. By linking to European

Catholicism at this precise historical moment, the healing in a sense flaunted America's new foreign policy of withdrawing into its own borders. Thus the Mattingly cure highlighted American Catholicism's transatlantic context during a formative moment.

The cure and responses to it crystallized fundamental debates within the early American church about its future direction and development. The events of 1824 helped push Catholicism into the shape it began to assume in the United States during the 1830s—that of multiple immigrant enclaves. The Mattingly miracle was the field on which the forces of continental Catholicism sparred with the Anglo-American "native" perspective over the formation of nineteenth-century American Catholicism. Ultimately, continental Catholicism largely prevailed, and the American Catholic Church became more alienated from its roots in the Maryland tradition of its English founders. With Catholicism's exposed rifts being played out in the aftermath of Ann Mattingly's miracle cure, the Protestant response to the cure can also be seen as a harbinger of a growing American anti-Catholicism that would take hold during the 1830s and broadly manifest about the time of Ann Mattingly's death in 1855. Furthermore, backlash against the miracle helped fuel sentiments that energized the Know-Nothing Party of the 1850s.

German Mysticism

An important context for the reception in the United States of Prince Hohenlohe's miracle working is not only religious, but also literary. While England, France, and Spain were dominant cultural forces in America, the German confederation, which existed from 1815 to 1866, also played a significant, though lesser, cultural role. The figure of the German mystic was familiar to early Americans through works such as those penned by the "Father of the American Novel," Charles Brockden Brown. German mysticism is explored in Brown's 1798 gothic thriller *Weiland: Or, The Transformation* and in folktales such as *Grimm's Fairy Tales.* The charismatic healer, Prince Hohenlohe, would have been a recognizable literary type of evil protagonist to Americans of this generation.

Folktales from the romantic German Black Forest first appeared in English in 1819 in the body of an article in the *Quarterly Review* by Francis Palgrave, father of the editor of the *Golden Treasury*. During 1821–1822, Edgar Taylor began publishing his translations of works by the Brothers Grimm in articles appearing in the *New Monthly Magazine and Literary Journal* under the title "German Popular and Traditional Literature." Like Prince Hohenlohe, the Brothers Grimm were from Bavaria, where folk magic and superstition thrived in the forests of southern Germany. George Cruikshank, who also drew a lampoon of Prince Hohenlohe for another British publication, was the illustrator.[2]

Despite the proscriptions of the Monroe Doctrine, the culture and ideas of Catholic Europe, including Germany, continued to cross-pollinate with early American culture, and it is reasonable to assume that the appearance of *Grimm's Fairy Tales* and the poems of such German writers as Johann Wolfgang von Goethe would have helped shape the reception of the Mattingly miracle, in which a German wonder worker cured a prominent citizen. Given such literary precedents, American readers may well have associated German mysticism with charlatanism, superstition, and gullibility.

A quarter century after Prince Gallitzin exorcised the demons from Adam Livingston's house in frontier Virginia, tales of Prince Hohenlohe, who healed the sick in partnership with a peasant farmer, began to circulate in the United States. The dramatic story of Princess Mathilde von Schwarzenberg's recovery was carried in print, in letters, and by word of mouth in American and British publications. The number of stories about Prince Hohenlohe before the 1824 cure is surprisingly substantial. As early as November 1, 1821, the *Charleston City Gazette and Commercial Daily Advertiser* ran a story dated July 7 of that year "from the French papers" about Prince Hohenlohe's triumphant return to Bamberg after his cure of the princess. The statement of Nanni Kemper, Mathilde's governess, was reprinted with this article. Bishop John England's Catholic publication *The United States Catholic Miscellany* also ran a story on October 9, 1822, about Mathilde's cure. On May 5, 1823, the *Alexandria Herald* in Virginia published a story about two Hohenlohe cures in England. News of cures in Dublin followed in November 1923 published in a newspaper in Ithaca, New York. On January 5, 1824, the *Catholic Miscellany* trumpeted cures in France and an attempted cure in Baltimore of a male mathematics professor, Mr. M. L. Chevigne. The next day, an announcement of a new book about the prince appeared in the *Boston Medical Intelligencer* and again in a Rhode Island paper in February 1824. Prince Hohenlohe was a familiar enough figure that just one month before Ann Mattingly's cure in Washington, D.C., the *Charleston City Gazette and Commercial Daily Advertiser* published a satirical piece, likely reprinted from the Dublin papers, called "Prince Hohenlohe Rivaled," which it expected would amuse its readers.[3]

Between September 13, 1821, and December 2, 1823, the *London Times,* which was available in the United States, ran at least ten articles about Prince Hohenlohe. As might be expected, they are informed by the same negative Protestant response that would be expressed after Mrs. Mattingly's cure. One writer stated, "regarding the pretended miracles of Prince Hohenlohe; the point is decided—decided to be gross and scandalous delusion—an impudent fraud, for the base purpose of degrading the human character, and creating rebellion not only against the empire of reason, but against the liberal institutions of all free countries." Wording such as this supported the notion of a reasoned Protestantism versus an irrational Catholicism. Unitarian readers in America might have heard of the prince via the pages of the *Monthly Repository of Theology and General Literature,* which in 1822 devoted several pages to mocking "Catholic Miracles in Germany." American periodicals such as the *Miscellaneous Cabinet* and the *New Monthly Magazine and Literary Journal* also published sarcastic articles about Hohenlohe miracles before the Mattingly cure.[4]

But the prince was not universally scorned in North America. In 1823, New York publisher James Costigan brought out an account of *Miracles Wrought by the Intersession of Prince Hohenlohe* that detailed the English healings of Mary Lalor, Mary Stuart, and Barbara O'Connor. Laudatory stories about the prince's healing powers in English and other languages were carried to Americans and to friends of the Carberys. The Carberys were a family of prominent citizens and devout Catholics. As such, they would have had access to reports from Europe in Catholic and secular presses about the miracles of Prince Hohenlohe and be well placed to petition for the delivery of Ann from her illness. Ann's sister Mary, a Carmelite nun at Portobacco, and her younger brother Joseph, a Jesuit priest, could have learned of Hohenlohe's works through religious networks. Stories of cures in monasteries in England, in Ireland, and on the European continent spread through religious and secular channels. At least one letter in the archives of the Visitation Monastery in Georgetown dated October 20, 1822, discusses an appeal to the prince for the healing of a "Mother Clare."[5]

The unusual conflation of local and federal government in Washington City inflated the national importance of incidents in the mayor's office and family. Hence, during the final months of Thomas Carbery's term as mayor in 1824, Washington City was riveted by news of his sister's miraculous cure.[6]

The Seeds of Controversy

During its foundational years, the American church had been deeply preoccupied with practical matters such as ecclesiastical organization and missionary work. The church struggled to attend to its basic institutional challenges, such as building parishes and training priests and nuns to staff them. This attempt to gain a foothold in the United States without a fully functioning organizational structure in place produced one hallmark of this age: lay trusteeism. Several states, especially in the South, actually prohibited the incorporation of religious bodies, so lay trustees, or wardens, stepped forward to help address the practical needs of establishing churches among scattered Catholic settlers and of ministering to them without sufficient numbers of clergy. Lay initiative seemed to provide a workable solution to the dilemma and was heartily endorsed by John Carroll, the first American bishop. But the lay trusteeism that John Carroll viewed as a building block for the American church had dangerous implications for episcopal authority—and implications for the reception of the Mattingly miracle.

Once a supply of additional American bishops began to be appointed, they encountered powerful lay trustees who were unwilling to relinquish the power they had come to enjoy. Lay trustees boldly claimed the right to appoint and dismiss their own pastors, though canon law vested that right solely in the hands of bishops. Influenced by the American Protestant tradition of congregationalism and the American political system of localism, lay trustees pressured bishops to bend to their demands. Early American bishops faced an American Catholic laity who had been raised in the atmosphere of anticlericalism brought to this nation by some European immigrants. European priests who were more at home in a traditional hierarchical church expressed discomfort with this American tendency toward self-government within local parishes. The Irish, especially, had a long history of lay control of church matters and also produced their share of fractious priests—priests unwilling to submit to authority, such as the renegade "Democritus," discussed later in this chapter, who criticized the handling of the Mattingly miracle by church officials in the pages of the *National Intelligencer.*

Archbishop Maréchal of Baltimore, a key figure in the Mattingly controversy, had conflicts with lay trustees in Virginia and South Carolina. Maréchal was typical of the first group of French Catholic leaders: learned, aristocratic exiles fleeing European libertarian democracies. These exiles collaborated with the Anglo-American establishment to try to keep church power in the hands of affluent Catholics in order to prevent the overspread of Irish Catholicism. The ascent of the lower-class Irish in the American church would, in the perceptions of the established Catholics, invite nativist attacks and fray the delicate intellectual and social ties with the American Protestant establishment that they had worked so hard to weave.[7]

The parish where the Carberys worshipped, St. Patrick's, is the oldest parish in the Federal City, founded in 1794 by John Carroll to provide a place of worship for the Irish stonemasons building the White House and the U.S. Capitol. The church was dedicated to Ireland's patron saint, Patrick, and Ann Mattingly's cure would come during March, the month of St. Patrick's feast. It was the first church of any denomination erected in the capital that, along with the city of Georgetown and the county of

Washington, would merge to form a single territorial government known as the District of Columbia in 1871. William W. Warner, in his book about Georgetown's history, notes that as members of Congress, senators, journalists, government officials, merchants, and distinguished visitors from all over the young republic descended on the new capital city, they did not find an alien "immigrant church" so often ascribed to urban Catholicism in the United States. Rather, they found well-to-do, educated, and civic-minded Catholics working in the highest circles of government, dedicated to the challenge of building the Capital City.[8]

When Ann and John Mattingly moved to the Federal City about 1805, Catholics had a strong foothold in Washington. For instance, the first mayor of Washington, Robert Brent, a Catholic, had been appointed by Thomas Jefferson in 1802 and held the position for a decade. James Hoban, a Catholic architect, designed the White House and other public buildings. One of the early presidents of Georgetown College, Giovanni Antonio Grassi, recorded the surprised reactions of visitors who observed Washington's urbane Catholics: "Is that the teaching of the Catholic church? Is that upright gentleman a Catholic? How different from the idea I had formed of it!" The fifth- and sixth-generation American Catholics encountered by visitors were not very different from themselves, a realization that Warner suggests had begun to effectively erode the cultural legacies of anti-Popery and Guy Fawkes Day brought from Europe by English-speaking settlers. Yet, the Mattingly miracle threatened to undermine the successful integration of Catholics into the life of the capital city and the nation and helped foster the emergence of an alternative tradition in American Catholicism: the immigrant tradition.[9]

Historian Thomas W. Spalding has called the kind of social and cultural engagement of American Catholics in Washington the "Maryland tradition," and it has several features that took seed in the imagination of the Catholic Calverts, Lords of Baltimore, and John Carroll: a "neutral state based upon the principles of religious freedom and separation of church and state," and an "ardent patriotism born of Revolutionary ferment, an appreciation of the democratic processes and structures these principles called forth, and a conviction that the new republic was destined to play a missionary, even messianic role, in promoting such principles, procedures, and structures." The Maryland tradition was ecumenical, with a "strong civic sense that found an outlet in public service." Influenced deeply by the French Sulpician order, the Maryland tradition embraced a "moderate Gallicanism" that privileged the needs of local American churches above those of the papacy and developed American-style autonomy from Rome.[10]

In 1799, tensions had arisen between two orders of priests in the United States, the Jesuits and the Sulpicians, over the founding of a rival institution to Georgetown College, the future St. Mary's College in Baltimore. Bishop John Carroll developed a mistrust of European Jesuits, writing in 1815 that they were too often not "discerning enough to estimate the difference between the American character; and that of the Countries, which they left." Carroll favored an approach more like that of Rev. William Matthews, the pastor of St. Patrick's, who immersed himself in the fabric of the Federal City, cofounding the city's first public library and serving on the school board. Both Carroll and Matthews preferred that the local church blend imperceptibly into the social fabric. The moderate Gallicanism of the Sulpicians provided for what historian Christopher Kauffman has called "the movement of the Holy Spirit in the *particular* national context rather than in the *centralized* authority structures of the papacy."[11]

With the ascension in 1816 of Carroll's successor, Archbishop Leonard Neale, who served for about a year and a half, the currents of ethnic discord were set in motion. Though Neale worked diligently to promote the Jesuits, the next archbishop, Ambrose Maréchal, was a Sulpician. By 1817, Catholicism had achieved respect and an unprecedented level of security in the nation as the inauguration of President James Monroe ushered in what would become known as the Era of Good Feelings. Catholic leaders shared this sense of "good feelings," and in October 1818, Maréchal reported to Rome: "All religions are tolerated here, and the laws of the Republic protect them all and most severely punish those who attempt to disturb the divine worship of any sect. And since religious liberty is the fundamental principle of the American Republic, there is no magistrate from the President to the

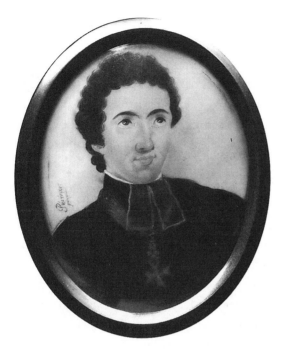

Miniature of Prince Alexander Hohenlohe that belonged to Ann Carbery Mattingly. Photo by John Holloway. Collection of Georgetown Visitation Monastery Archives.

least official, who can with impunity molest Catholics in the least way." The archbishop's report is a snapshot of a halcyon moment for American Catholicism, but forces were already conspiring to undo it. In the midst of identifying an idyllic period in American Catholicism, Maréchal prophetically underscored some of the internal currents that would help dismantle it: "The only danger that blocks the path of our most holy religion, consists in the internal dissentions which divide the faithful against each other."[12]

As the star of the Sulpicians rose under Archbishop Maréchal, the tide turned for the Jesuits, and the "internal dissentions" the archbishop feared would begin to rock the American church to its core. In December 1818, a pamphlet called "Letter to Thomas Jefferson" was sent to governors and legislatures of all the states. Written by a Catholic, possibly Dr. John F. Oliviera Fernandez, in response to Maréchal's attempts to rein in the power of trustees and clergy at Norfolk, Virginia, and Charleston, South Carolina, the letter was one obvious sign of the downward turn. The anonymous writer warned that American Jesuits were ambitious and greedy and urged elected officials to "limit the power of foreign governments with our territory," a reference to the preponderance of French-born American bishops, but also a foreshadowing of the nativist movements that would arise in the 1830s. The battles over the Mattingly miracle would make these growing fissures evident to the nation.[13]

"News of Supernatural Facts"

As Mrs. Mattingly's health failed over seven years, her pastor, William Matthews, and two Jesuit priests with ties to Georgetown, Anthony Kohlmann (1771–1836), a native of Alsace, and Stephen Dubuisson (1786–1864), who had been born in Santo Domingo in the Caribbean, discussed the idea of following Prince Hohenlohe's directions for a cure of Ann Mattingly. These Jesuits were well known in the Catholic community. Kohlmann had been appointed vicar general of the diocese of New York in 1808. In one of the stranger and oft-challenged legends of U.S. history, it is said that Kohlmann and Benedict Fenwick had been called to the deathbed of the atheist Thomas Paine in 1809. Paine had reportedly hoped the priests might administer some medical assistance, but when they attempted the salvation of his immortal soul, the dying man raged and cursed them out of the room.[14]

In 1813, Kohlmann made legal history in New York by winning an important court challenge for the American Catholic Church, successfully defending the seal of confession in a controversial case. The vicar had been instrumental in restoring stolen goods to a robbery victim, who then demanded in court that the priest reveal the name of the culprit in the crime. Kohlmann refused on the grounds that his information had been received under the seal of confession. The case was brought before the New York Court of General Sessions, where, after a trial, the judge and future governor, DeWitt Clinton, ruled in Kohlmann's favor.

In 1817, Kohlmann assumed the presidency of Georgetown College after the departure to Europe of Giovanni "John" Grassi. Kohlmann's administration is generally considered a setback for the college because of his "chronic volatility and his chronic difficulties with Anglo-Americans." Georgetown historian R. Emmett Curran bluntly termed it a "disaster." The students chafed under the strict discipline that Kohlmann imposed and, in 1818, even plotted to murder Stephen Dubuisson, who had been given the job of enforcing the college's rules. The faculty battled over curriculum along ethnic lines, with continental Jesuits opposing Anglo-Americans, or "native" Jesuits, who favored a broader range of academic areas.[15]

Not surprisingly, these are the same rival camps that were identified by historian Thomas Murphy, who defined native Jesuits as those who were raised in the British Isles and "continentalist" Jesuits as those who came from the European mainland. Kohlmann and the continental Jesuits were also quite aggressive in their attempts to convert non-Catholic students, resulting in some tempests with Protestant parents. With Kohlmann's departure in 1820, the college struggled to rebuild, but the conflicts between competing educational philosophies, continental and native, came to a head after the Mattingly miracle, and several faculty left the college.[16]

Differences over many issues, including property ownership, continued between Archbishop Maréchal and the Jesuits, similar to what had flared up between St. Patrick's William Matthews and members of the Society of Jesus. Maréchal traveled to Rome to press his views and appealed to Cardinal Ercole Consalvi, acting prefect of the propaganda, during the same period in 1822 that Consalvi was dealing with the Hohenlohe controversy in Germany. In a papal brief dated June 23, 1822, the Vatican ordered that the Jesuits defer to the decisions of the archbishop and surrender the two-thousand-acre White Marsh plantation in Prince George's County, an estate they had held since 1729 and one of the earliest Catholic missions in the American colonies, to the archbishop's control. The Jesuits responded by filing a claim that the U.S. government would not allow the alienation of property ordered by a foreign body, the Holy See. In 1824, the year of Mrs. Mattingly's miraculous cure, Kohlmann was superior of the Jesuit plantation at White Marsh and was still at odds with Maréchal over its control. Trustees of St. Patrick's complained of "the intrigues of disobedient clergymen and . . . impious and turbulent laymen" in their parish, a seeming reference to their assistant pastor, Stephen Dubuisson.[17]

Dubuisson's family had fled Santo Domingo during a revolution in 1793, taking refuge in France. There, Dubuisson had joined the army and served as a staff officer of Napoleon until he resigned in protest over the emperor's imprisonment of Pius VII in 1809, shortly before the emperor's Paris wedding gala went up in flames in 1810. The same year that Ann Mattingly had moved with her children into her brother's house, 1815, Dubuisson had been ordained a Jesuit. His contemplative aspirations made him ill-suited to the role of disciplinarian at Georgetown College, and the 1818 plot against his life unnerved him. In 1821, while an assistant pastor to Matthews at St. Patrick's, he wrote to Archbishop Maréchal to complain of his supervisor: "Rev. Mr. Matthews uses for internments, and likewise for baptisms, the English translations of the Roman Ritual instead of the Latin Original. . . . This is quite contrary to the universal practice of the Catholic Church."[18] No response from the archbishop has been preserved, and the practice continued, but it is likely that Matthews knew of or suspected this breach of loyalty.

The two principal actors, then, in the Mattingly miracle, Dubuisson and Matthews, had very different views about church practices at St. Patrick's. Dubuisson had read the 1822 *Cures Miraculeuses Obtenues par les prières du Prince Abbé de Hohenlohe en 1821 et 1822* (Miraculous Cures Obtained by the Prayers of Prince Father de Hohenlohe in 1821 and 1822) and had already written to Prince Hohenlohe on behalf of other sick Catholics in Washington. He had been following stories of European cures in the French newspaper *L'Ami de la Religion*. When Kohlmann, his former teacher, asked him to write to the prince specifically on behalf of Mrs. Mattingly, he was at first reluctant, since the prince had not responded to his earlier communications; but in January 1824, he again wrote to the healer and would later formally request permission to proceed with the novena from Archbishop Maréchal. On February 6, Dubuisson received a letter from William Beschter, a German Jesuit who had been composing the petitions for Baltimore parishioners with Rev. John Tessier. Beschter quoted from a letter from the prince and appended a postscript, "à toutes les prières pour guérison un bon paysan nommé Martin Michel est prié de joindre les siennes s'il faisait les mêmes cures avant le Prince de Hohenlohe [during all the prayers for healing a good country farmer is asked to join his own prayers with those of Prince Hohenlohe]." Participation of Martin Michel, the "bon paysan," in the American cures, however, was prevented by the farmer's death on February 29, 1824, the day before the novena began in Washington.[19]

Archbishop Maréchal gave Dubuisson his permission for the novena but reminded the St. Patrick's priest of the Catholic prohibition against offering Mass in the sick chamber and expressed doubt that a strict regimen would be necessary in order to "say Mass in union with the Prince." In his letter, the archbishop stated that priests were not bound to say Mass "sooner or later according to the difference of Longitude between the place they live in and Bamberg Because—1st the French letter or paragraph is printed and manifestly destined for Priests living in neighbouring Countries where they can without inconvenience say Mass at 9 OClock or a little sooner or later 2nd. Because if Mass were to be said by the Priest at the precise hour, The Prince says it himself, in many Countries Mass should be said at midnight or before. 3rd. Because the Prince is in deed habitually in Bamberg but moves frequently from place to place. When he wrote to Rev. Mr. Tessier he was in Hungary. Who can tell where he will be on the 10th of next month—no body I am sure."[20] Though Maréchal demonstrated an awareness of the problematic logistics of saying Mass in union with Prince Hohenlohe, the European Jesuits in Washington were determined to precisely abide by Hohenlohe's directions.

The archbishop also issued this caution: "I have certainly no objection to your performing the acts of Devotion prescribed by Prince Hohenlohe. Myself on the 10th will join you my prayers to yours—but let no noise be made about it lest impious men should take from thence an occasion of ridiculing or blaspheming our Holy Religion." Maréchal would soon take a similar position arguing for an avoidance of scandal after the miracle, writing, "news of supernatural facts, are generally calculated to excite in the mind of the people, very strong sentiments which often prompt them to go beyond the limits traced by enlightened piety and even ordinary prudence." The Sulpician Maréchal, then, cautioned moderation over enthusiasm, in keeping with his sense of the enlightened rationalism of his adopted nation. Like other French aristocrats in the church hierarchy, such as Bishop John Cheverus of Boston, Maréchal enjoyed a good rapport with Protestants and feared that too much enthusiasm about miracles might revive the dormant anti-Popery sentiment that had been buried through the cooperation of the French during the American Revolution.[21]

Dubuisson began to plan a set of devotional rituals according to Prince Hohenlohe's instructions beginning on Monday, March 1, 1824. Three sick people in addition to Mrs. Mattingly were included on the prayer list: William Boone, Mary Noyes, and Eliza Wimsatt. The novena prayers were the litany of the holy name of Jesus, specified by the prince, and other prayers, including "Lord Jesus! May thy name be glorified," to be uttered at sunrise by the approximately two hundred friends and relatives who joined in the devotion. Despite the archbishop's dismissal of the need to time the Mass exactly with the longitude of the prince's location, Dubuisson began his Mass at St. Patrick's at about 2:00 A.M. on the morning of Wednesday, March 10. Kohlmann offered Mass at the Georgetown College chapel beginning at 3:30 A.M. Tessier joined them in prayer in Baltimore, as did Ann's brother Joseph Carbery, and it is possible that other priests did as well. Two of the petitioners attended Dubuisson's service at St. Patrick's, but according to Matthews, "no change took place" in their health. The other petitioner and Mrs. Mattingly were too ill to attend a service, so the Eucharist was brought to them after the Mass.[22]

When Dubuisson arrived at Thomas Carbery's home, Mrs. Mattingly's sight and hearing were failing. A small towel was placed under her chin. She tried to adjust it, but her arm was paralyzed. She had already taken more than 350 drops of laudanum that day for pain. Before he administered Communion, Dubuisson read excerpts from Prince Hohenlohe's letter to the dying Mrs. Mattingly: "Be then animated with a strong faith, which excludes all doubts and hesitation, with a truly filial unlimited confidence in the promises of a Father, whose goodness and mercy are infinite as his omnipotence. But let us remember, that in asking to be delivered from the evils which afflict us, we ought to desire it principally in order to be in a state to serve him better, and to fulfill more faithfully the duties of our stations." With this admonition to be faithful and use the divine gift in service to the church, Dubuisson administered the Eucharist—which instantly healed Mrs. Mattingly. The stunned witnesses would later testify to that moment in affidavits and certificates published in the late spring of 1824.[23]

In the midst of the excitement in the mayor's house after the healing, Dubuisson left to tend to the other petitioner who had been too ill to attend Mass; the historical record is silent on whether or not that cure occurred. Before daybreak, Dubuisson had sent the happy news about Mrs. Mattingly's cure to his superior at Georgetown, the Reverend Francis Dzierozynski. "Miracle! Reverend and Dear Father Superior," he wrote. "Mrs. Mattingly was suddenly relieved from all pains this morning at 4:15 about seven minutes after receiving communion. She immediately was able to get up and return thanks on her knees. Lord Jesus! Thy name be glorified." He then requested permission to hire a horse and ride to Baltimore to personally deliver the news to the archbishop. In his saddlebag, he carried a euphoric letter from Rev. William Matthews, in which the pastor called Mrs. Mattingly "the most perfect model of human perfection I know or ever expect to see," for the fortitude with which she had borne her illness, and wrote of his excitement over her "miraculous & instantaneous cure." The next day, the bells of Georgetown College rang out the joyous news of Mrs. Mattingly's healing, and Stephen Dubuisson drafted an ecstatic letter to Prince Hohenlohe to tell him the news. Rev. Tessier's response in his diary was more measured: "A superb day. I planted some small onions. M. Dubuisson came to tell us that there took place in Washington a great miracle due to the intercession of Prince Hohenlohe. The Archbishop intends to go there, to investigate."[24]

Archbishop Maréchal deliberated for two days before responding to Matthews. In a long and carefully considered rejoinder, he acknowledged that a miracle was a potential inducement to conversions and the strengthening of Catholicism in the United States. Aware that the highly favorable place of Catholics had eroded from the halcyon days of five years before, the archbishop expressed deep concern that the event might generate excitement that could be harmful to the situation of the American church. Since, as he had pointed out, "supernatural facts" can "excite in the mind of the people, very strong sentiments," "it is the duty of secondary pastors and a portion of mine to moderate and guide the popular emotion how laudable however it may be in its source and principles. Permit me then Rev. and dear sir to trace you some rules of conduct in the present and important circumstance in which you are placed."[25]

Maréchal then outlined five steps for Matthews to follow: (1) the expressions of gratitude for the cure should be limited to the family and the parish; (2) prudence should dictate what is published in the newspapers; (3) affidavits should be collected to document the cure; (4) Protestant witnesses and respectable Catholics should be called; and (5) copies of the certificates should be sent to him. The archbishop had hoped to maintain a measure of control over the event but could not have foreseen the intense interest it generated. During the first two days after the cure, March 10 and 11, five hundred visitors came to see Mrs. Mattingly. Mayor Thomas Carbery, likely overwhelmed by these numbers, wrote to the archbishop, pleading for direction: "We shall not make public this affair, till we see or hear from you, which I trust for the honour and glory of the Catholic cause will be soon." Kohlmann informed a fellow Jesuit that the city was "electrified." A few days later, he reported that Mrs. Mattingly had received not five hundred, but one thousand visitors on the day of her cure, and more than two thousand the next—and she shook hands with all of them, smiling, laughing, and conversing. Another priest compared the exhilaration in Washington to that in Jerusalem upon the arrival of the Magi. The urbane and sophisticated Maréchal was acutely aware of how these stories would play in the hands of those who wished to harm Catholicism.[26]

As soon as the excitement took hold of the Federal City, rumors began to fly, and, as the archbishop had feared, some began to mock the Catholics. A story circulated at the Navy Yard that Dubuisson had broken his leg on the way to Baltimore and that the Archbishop had raised his hand over the fractured leg and said, 'Arise, Dubuisson, thy leg is cured, and walk home'" Another tale that made its way through the city was that Rev. Anthony Kohlmann had converted half the town of Annapolis by preaching on the miracle there. A gothic version appeared in Philadelphia's *National Gazette and Literary Register* and the *New York Statesman* ten days after the miracle. In it, the writer described a scene in which a priest, who seemed to some to be a caricature of Kohlmann, regaled his listeners with the tale of Mrs. Mattingly's cure: "We were seated in a group around the Father Confessor, near the window. At the commencement of the miraculous tale enough twilight and beams of the moon came through a solitary casement to render the form and features of the venerable man half visible. He wore glasses and a black cap upon his head. At the most solemn part of the story, a breath of wind or the unobserved hand of a servant, closed the shutter, and we were left in total darkness, while the reverend father pursued and finished his narration. It was a scene I would not have lost for all the pleasures of the winter."[27]

Like the literary figures in *Grimm's Fairy Tales* that underlay some of the reception of the German miracle worker, so elements of the gothic made their way into the reporting of the event. The metaphorical connection of the miracle to either of these genres would arouse American skepticism. Alarmed by the fabrications and mindful of the warning of the archbishop, Matthews discouraged plans for Mrs. Mattingly to walk from her home to St. Patrick's for Mass, as well as other ideas for promoting the miracle. On March 31, 1824, a frustrated Maréchal lashed out at Stephen Dubuisson for his lack of circumspection and particularly noted that Dubuisson had ignored his instructions to not try to time the Masses in Washington with those in Europe.[28]

The Protestant Response

Puritans and other Protestant settlers carried to the United States an anti-Popery sentiment most often associated with the English tradition in Great Britain. While many negative responses to the prince, especially, do not self-identify with a particular Protestant denomination, there is a recognizable pattern of satire and mockery that one readily associates with the English tradition of anti-Popery. This anti-Catholic theme can be seen in the numerous publications about the Mattingly miracle and the prince that appeared in the United States after the event.

One way to trace the Protestant response to the miracle is in the numerous newspaper and magazine articles that appeared beginning in March 1824, and especially in the many American reprints of unfriendly British publications. News of Mrs. Mattingly's dramatic healing was reprinted in newspapers along the eastern seaboard. For instance, nine days after the event, on March 19, an article appeared in the *Salem Gazette* in Massachusetts that referenced Hohenlohe's by then well-known European cures and announced, "it appears that the supernatural power of this Prince has found its way into our country." The *Gazette* reprinted an article that had been published in the *New York Statesman* titled "Washington, March 10, 1824." A day later, March 20, the same story was reprinted in Portsmouth, New Hampshire, and on March 22 in newspapers in Baltimore and Boston. By March 23, the story had spread to two more papers in Providence, Rhode Island, and in Richmond, Virginia, and a follow-up article appeared in the Salem newspaper. By the end of March 1824, articles about the Mattingly miracle appeared in newspapers in Charleston, South Carolina; Haverhill, Massachusetts; Cooperstown, New York; Danville, Vermont; and New London, Connecticut. Though carried by couriers on horseback, the story had, to use a twenty-first-century expression, gone viral.[29]

Of a sample of eighteen extant articles published between March 19 and March 31, 1824, only two were positive. The *Richmond Enquirer* published one such piece on March 26, reprinting a letter written by a gentleman of the city of Washington on March 13, 1824, who proclaimed: "The presidential question is at this moment thrown completely out of view, by a miracle wrought by Prince Hohenlohe, of whom you have no doubt, ere this time, repeatedly heard of or read. This wonder, which has absorbed the attention of everybody in this metropolis, for the last three days, was performed by the Prince on a very respectable lady nearly allied to our worthy mayor." The story, then, was deemed as newsworthy as the race for the presidency. Nine of the eighteen articles were neutral in their presentation of the story, and seven, or 39 percent, were negative. The *Essex Register* of March 29, which noted that its editor was Catholic, reprinted an editorial from the *Edinburgh Review* that stated, "We will venture to assert that there is not one rational Catholic, who, in his cooler moments, does not regret the attempt now making to palm such gross impositions upon the world"; it then raised concerns that the miracle story could contribute to sectarian strife in the United States. This is the view that would come to be shared by some of the native Jesuits, who feared that the story would compromise American Catholicism. A satirical piece reprinted from a newspaper in Belfast, Ireland, related the prince's miraculous assistance with the capture of a mouse, which it called "the greatest miracle ever wrought by that wonder-working divine." In Cooperstown, New York, the *Watch-Tower* of April 29 headlined its article, "The Days of St. Patrick and the Snakes Returned!"[30]

An article titled "Humbug" that originally ran in the *National Advertiser* might in part explain this spate of publications. The writer editorializes, "The public in general are so thirsty after anecdotes of this kind, that a newspaper is thought to be dull without them." But it is likely anti-Popery sentiment that helped make these stories so widely circulated. In addition to mocking European cures, there were attempts to undermine the power of the miracle by printing false reports about Mrs. Mattingly, such as "From the Evening Post," reprinted in the *Saratoga Sentinel:* "It is, perhaps, not generally known, that the lady said to have been recently cured at Washington of a deadly disease, by the miraculous prayers of Prince Hohenlohe, shortly afterward relapsed into her former ill state of health."[31]

Another aspect of the story that took on a magnified importance was the mayoral election of June 1824, which Mayor Carbery lost. The reportage carried a distinctly anti-Catholic tone. The election came on the heels of both the miracle and a series of articles in a southern publication, the *Mount Zion Missionary.* This publication raised the specter that Catholicism was essentially incompatible with democracy, averring, "Republicanism and Catholicism bear no affinity in any one single relation, nor can they ever cor-

dially unite in character." While these words were not specifically directed
at the mayoral election in Washington, Catholic historian Peter Guilday
cites this slogan as a harbinger of the brewing national question of whether
Roman Catholicism could ever be compatible with American democracy.[32]

In its gleeful reporting of Mayor Carbery's defeat, some of the press
linked the Mattingly miracle to politics. A Boston newspaper gloated over
the news of Carbery's defeat in the mayoral election: "We have been informed that this extraordinary cure has caused a certain religious excitement or *revival* at Washington, and has defeated the re-election of Mr.
Thomas Carberry [*sic*], the brother of Mrs. Mattingly, to the office of mayor.
We live indeed in an age of wonders, and pregnant with events—but really,
but of all the reasons that could be adduced to justify the dismission of a
man from office, the most extraordinary reason is to dismiss him because
he permits this wonderful cure to take place under his roof." Underlying
this quotation is the mainstream Protestant position that the age of miracles
had ended. The writer of the passage satirically links the mayor's defeat
with a miraculous event. Several other newspapers echoed the sentiment
that the miracle had cost Carbery the election. If, indeed, the miracle did
affect the election because of latent anti-Catholic feeling, there would be an
irony in worrying that Catholics could not sufficiently separate from their
religious convictions to participate in democracy.[33]

In addition to newspaper reports, magazine articles and pamphlets
also addressed the controversial cure. Protestant backlash to the Mattingly
miracle is illustrated, for instance, in an essay published in the *Washington Theological Repertory* on April 1, 1824. The author, writing under the
pseudonym Chrysostom, concluded that "men of reading, reflection, and
sense, will laugh at their [the Catholics'] pretensions: and feel indignant,
that in this age and country, an attempt should be made to impose upon
the credulity of the people, by a branch of that body which forged and
riveted, and are now trying to rivet again, the chains of ignorance and superstition under which the people of Europe have so long been groaning;
but they may be assured there is a description of people even in America,
as ready to be caught by miraculous pretence, as ever bowed at the shrine

of *Thomas a Becket.*" This reference to the archbishop of Canterbury, who was assassinated in 1170 for defying King Henry II, links the Mattingly miracle to ancient struggles between church and state in England and sets the stage for debate of the same issues in the United States. The reference to the alleged "chains of ignorance and superstition" of the Catholic Church is deliberately contrasted to American ideals of freedom and rationalism. Such terminology had many implications during a period when the topic of slavery was becoming a subject of national debate. The editor of the *Theological Repertory* was the Reverend William Hawley, of St. John's Episcopal Church in Washington, who would become more deeply embroiled in the controversy as the summer stretched on.[34]

The tone of much of this anti-Catholic discourse was drawn from the British model. Another journal, the *Reformer* of May 1, 1824, announced, "The present seems to be the age of wonders and (lying) miracles," and in July it called Prince Hohenlohe a "pious mountebank." Numerous articles and stories culled from British publications were reprinted in the United States as well, highly unfavorable to the prince and alluding to the question of whether miracles could occur in the modern era. The pamphlet skirmishes escalated in May 1824, when the *Orthodox Journal* in London published "An Examination of a Protestant's Objections to the Popish Miracle Lately Wrought in America," which was a response to a scathing letter published about the Mattingly miracle in another English publication, the *Preston Chronicle.* The headline was "The Popish Miracle," and the writer signed his name "A 'Protestant.'"[35]

The *Preston Chronicle* had previously published an account of the miracle by Rev. Kohlmann, and a letter of response from "A Protestant" was reprinted in its entirety. He began by making this objection: "On reading it over, I found that, as usual, the individual upon whom the miracle was wrought, is a *Papist.* These priests and princes can work no miracles upon us poor Protestants; all their miracles are wrought upon *Papists,* by *Papists,* with *Papists,* for *Papists:* indeed, it is a piece of Popery from beginning to end. Are they so bigotted they will not work? or are they so orthodox, they cannot? Or what? Excuse my skepticism, Mr. Editor, but this part of the story looks suspicious, really." "A Protestant" continues his polemic: "I was also struck with the place in which this miracle was wrought—America. Surely, all the diseased in Europe could not be cured, so that Prince Hohenlohe's powers were wasting out. But a great distance is a great thing in these cases, Mr. Editor. Excuse my skepticism. Like quack doctors, their cures have always been wrought at some considerable distance." He then asks, "And who is the Rev. A. Kohlman [*sic*], of Maryland? Nobody knows? . . . It would puzzle anybody to tell whether the Popish priests have made Christianity more detestable to infidels by their cruelties, or ridiculous by their absurdities." The mocking tone becomes almost a parody of the contemporary British anti-Catholic response, while attempting to undermine the significance of the Washington miracle.[36]

The mockery associated with anti-Popery from Great Britain continued to inform the Protestant response in the United States for several years after the event. Five years later, Prince Hohenlohe was still in the news, as the *Salem Gazette* printed a story in 1829 in which a Mr. Wolff reported that not only was Prince Alexander Hohenlohe a drunk, but he was antipapal, blasphemous, and lascivious. In 1834, ten years after the Mattingly miracle, at least four newspapers published a satiric account of the prince's giving up on miracle cures after accidentally overlengthening a woman's leg because of a calculation error. These articles, followed by two more reprints in the *Ladies' Companion* and the *Baltimore Literary and Religious Magazine*, appeared in the months just before and after the burning of the Ursuline Convent in Charlestown, Massachusetts, an event fueled by gender anxiety, ethnic strife, and religious intolerance that remains one of the most notorious acts of anti-Catholic violence of the time. Such publications show a visceral Protestant reaction to the miraculous cure of Ann Mattingly as long as ten years after the event and suggest that the story indeed played a role in the rising anti-Catholicism of the 1830s.[37]

"Friend of Truth"

The most extensive attack on the Mattingly miracle was published in July 1824, under the pseudonym Friend of Truth, in response to published affidavits about the miracle. The forty-one-page pamphlet was called "The Washington Miracle Refuted; or, a Review of the Rev. William Matthew's Pamphlet. By a Friend of Truth." Georgetown publisher James C. Dunn was the printer. The identity of the author has long been a subject of speculation, with most of the suspicion falling on the Jesuit Thomas C. Levins. However, in the notes Stephen Dubuisson made in preparation for refuting the pamphlet, he also names another suspect: "Hawley." Linguistic and other evidence indeed suggests that Rev. William Hawley, of St. John's Episcopal Church, was "Friend of Truth."[38]

Hawley was part of a group of Protestant Episcopal clergy who printed several attacks on the Roman Catholic Church published in the *Theological Repertory*. John England replied to this onslaught with a series of essays in the *Catholic Miscellany* during the same period of 1824–1825 called "Letters of Various Misrepresentations of the Catholic Religion," specifically addressed to Hawley. In these, England objects to, among other things, Hawley's insinuations that the United States is a Protestant country. During this raging print war, Hawley replied, "A Roman Catholic can be *in principle* a faithful subject of a Protestant government, only when an *unfaithful subject* of the Pope." The theme of Catholicism being incompatible with republicanism, then, is amplified in Hawley's writings. In July 1824, Hawley also took direct aim at his Catholic neighbors in Washington by attacking the Mattingly miracle and Prince Hohenlohe in a pamphlet written under the pseudonym Friend of Truth. The pamphlet savages the priests Stephen Dubuisson, Anthony Kohlmann, and William Matthews for their participation in the miracle and Archbishop Maréchal for his reticence over it. Friend of Truth's most vehement attacks are directed at the person he calls "Bishop Hohenlohe," though in 1824, the prince had not yet been named a bishop. Significantly, the essay opens with a quotation of St. Chrysostom, the pen name used in Hawley's satire in the *Theological*

Repertory: "Once it was known by miracles, who were true Christians and who false; but now the power of working miracles is wholly taken away, the pretence of it, is to be found among those who pretend to be Christians." The linguistic style of this article is also very similar to that of the article from the *Theological Repertory* of April 1824 already examined. Friend of Truth employs the same metaphor of slavery used in that article, writing, "None but a resident in those districts where the reason and free thought of the people, have been long exposed to the dominion under which the mental faculties of every *true* Papist *must* be enslaved; can accurately estimate the form with which miraculous presentations, like those so abundant in every page of Roman Catholic history, must strike upon the credulity and superstition of the multitude." This language echoes the imagery of chains and enslavement found in the April essay.[39]

Another linguistic parallel to Hawley's earlier work can be seen in a reference to "Thomas A Becket, Archbishop of Canterbury," which develops the accusation from the April article that the head of St. Thomas, which had been preserved in Canterbury as a Catholic relic and visited by thousands of pilgrims, was, he charges, "the head-piece of some poor, forgotten monk, and that the scull [*sic*] of St. Thomas had all the while [been] enjoying a sweet tranquility in his own grave."[40] These parallels in imagery and language strongly lead to the conclusion that Hawley is the author of the pamphlet. In its entirety, the pamphlet takes on each detail of *A Collection of Affidavits and Certificates, Relative to the Wonderful Cure of Mrs. Ann Mattingly, Which Took Place in the City of Washington, D.C. on the Tenth of March, 1824,* which had been published in late May 1824.

Friend of Truth mocks the two-month delay in publishing the affidavits and the shift from calling the event a "miracle" to merely a "wonderful cure." After the wait and toned-down representation of the event as a miracle, the writer declares that the pamphlet was "so much like the birth of a mouse from the parturient labours of a mountain, that I am sure no sensible Catholic can help mortification at the event." He mocks the secrecy with which the plans for the cure were undertaken, satirizing it as a "chamber" or "midnight" miracle." He attacks the timing of the miracle of sometime between 2:00 and 4:30 A.M., claiming that it did not take place simultaneously with Prince Hohenlohe's morning Mass in Germany and stating that, for Catholics apparently, "a miss is as good as a mile."[41]

Careful not to attack Mrs. Mattingly directly, which would be unchivalrous, he charges that her own affidavit shows she did not follow the prince's directions to actively believe that a cure was possible. Mrs. Mattingly, he states, by her own admission, had "calmly and without agitation of mind, awaited the final close of [her] earthly miseries." How, he asks, does this comply with the prince's explicit directions to have "an unrestricted confidence of being favorably heard"? Friend of Truth attacked everything about the miracle, from the "*seraphic* Kohlman [*sic*]" to "our modern Thaumaturgus, the long-fingered Hohenlohe," in a concerted attempt to undermine the validity of the miracle affidavits.[42]

The voice of the writer, in the sharp-tongued tradition of Jonathan Swift, drips with scorn and sarcasm, and he dissects the affidavits point by point. He scrutinizes the chronology of the events and the statements of the witnesses, ridiculing not only the priests, but Mrs. Mattingly's friends and family members as well. "This cure of Mrs. Mattingly, therefore, was but a chance shot of the Prince," Friend of Truth declares. He continues: "Like a child shooting into a flock at random and killing one bird, or like a quack doctor who publishes to the world a host of certificates setting forth the wonderful nature of a single cure, but forgetting to mention the thousand cases in which his medicine has failed; so have our Priests of Washington trumpeted forth their single instance of success, without having the candour to inform us of the many patients in their beds. Did the Apostles perform such miracles? Did they ever fail? Might not any one in Christendom, had he the effrontery of the Prince, be just as successful as he?" Friend of Truth goes on to discuss the difference between the clear and apparent miracles of Jesus and this murky Washington miracle.[43]

Friend of Truth also notes that petitions for Mrs. Mattingly's cure had originally been drawn up in 1823 and mocks the delay of more than a year in sending the petition to the prince for action while Mrs. Mattingly languished. Thomas Carbery is mercilessly skewered for being asleep in a nearby room when his sister was miraculously cured. But Friend of Truth saves his concluding venom for Prince Hohenlohe, reprinting unfavorable reports about the prince supplied to him "by a gentleman of Maryland who has a regular correspondent in the part of Germany where Hohenlohe has been operating." Friend of Truth concludes with a statement of a citizen of Bavaria who asserts: "My opinion, and also that of [the] thinking part of the Catholics and Protestants is, that he is far from being a true messenger of God. He has been made a dupe of by designing men, in consequence of which a serious disturbance has arisen, and if he had not been obliged to retreat, I would not have been surprised if a revolution had ensued." With this warning, Hawley, as Friend of Truth, connected the Washington miracle to his position stated in his other writings that Catholic doings are incompatible with national peace.[44]

"A Great Deal of Trouble": Dissention within the Catholic Church

After the publication of Hawley's pamphlet in July 1824, Bishop England responded with indignation, fuming: "We have read the refutation, yet! The refutation! Got through the entire 41 pages and what shall we say!"[45] But while Catholics had to contend with the vexing problems fueled by the Protestant reception of the miracle, a more serious and damaging split had arisen among various camps in Catholic Washington immediately after Ann Mattingly's cure. Two different perspectives may be traced in the Catholic reception to the miracle: that held by the continental Jesuit enthusiasts, such as Stephen Dubuisson, Anthony Kohlmann, William Beschter, Francis Dzierozynski, and Brother Joseph Mobberly, and that held by the moderate natives, which included the pastor of St. Patrick's, Rev. William Matthews; the Sulpician Archbishop Maréchal; John Tessier; and the English and American Jesuits such as Georgetown President Enoch Fenwick and Roger Baxter. Thomas C. Levins, who denounced the promotion of the miraculous event under the pen name Democritus, though he had an affinity with the moderate natives, took the more drastic step of airing these differences in a national newspaper. Irish-born Bishop John England, with his additional investigation of the miracle beginning in 1826 and culminating with a second publication in 1830 of affidavits attesting to the miracle, would with some degree of success manage to bring together an enthusiasm for modern miracles based on logical and rational evidence.

Immediately after the cure, reports abounded that the Federal City was abuzz with rumors and excitement, but Rev. Kohlmann's enthusiasm could barely be contained, as demonstrated by his letter to a New York lawyer published in the *Baltimore Federal Gazette* seventeen days after the miracle. "The Metropolis of America is moved," he wrote, "as Jerusalem formerly was at the arrival of the three wise men. It is in a transport of admiration and religious awe, and nothing can be thought or spoken of but the astonishing and splendid prodigy, which JESUS CHRIST, the Eternal Son of God, and most amiable Saviour of mankind, had been pleased to work, in the capital of America, and in sight of our national councils." The letter then relates the details of Ann Mattingly's dramatic cure, and Kohlmann adds: "All those that were there at the moment of her receiving the holy communion, and those that were acquainted with the horrid martyrdom which she suffered during six years, solemnly declare that they consider her miraculous restoration like unto, and equal to, the resuscitation of Lazarus from the grave, and that, to restore such a diseased, corrupted, and corroded frame, in a perfect state of health, required nothing less than the same creative power which had made her at first." Kohlmann creates a deliberate link to the biblical tradition of miracles, which is in direct contrast to the prevailing mainstream Protestant view of the time that the age of miracles ended in the early Christian era. His tone is triumphal and confrontational in asserting Catholicism as the true religion. Kohlmann's hyperbole exemplified the continental enthusiast camp and seemed to push native Jesuits and Sulpicians to respond. It was the beginning of serious and public dissention in the ranks of Washington Catholics.[46]

Rev. Matthews, a moderate in the Maryland tradition, tried to quell some of the exuberance by inserting a simple notice in the newspapers, such as the one that appeared in the *National Intelligencer* and *Baltimore Advertiser* at the end of March 1824:

As various, and in some instances, contradictory reports are circulated in the public prints relative to an extraordinary cure, effected in the person of one of my congregation, calculated to make an erroneous impression on the mind of persons at a distance, I have considered it as a deference due to the public from me, as Pastor of the Congregation to give an brief and correct statement of the occurrence. The simple fact is this—Mrs. Ann Mattingly, who has been, for the six years past, afflicted with a most painful internal disease, which resisted medicine and baffled the skill of the physician, was at an early hour on Wednesday morning, the 10th instant, after receiving holy communion, instantaneously healed, and restored to perfect health, which she has continued to enjoy since this date. She resides with her brother, Captain Carbery, the Mayor of this City.[47]

With this letter, Matthews was trying to follow the Archbishop Maréchal's directions for guiding the popular emotion.

At Maréchal's suggestion, Matthews proceeded to have the affidavits drawn up, but he privately expressed growing discomfort with the zeal of Dubuisson and Kohlmann in promoting the miracle. His full motives cannot be deciphered from this historical distance, but he was a voice of moderation, trying to keep the response to the miracle contained. In near exasperation, Matthews wrote to the archbishop about the planned collection of testimony: "I represented to Mr. Carbery and others the impropriety of introducing extraneous matter—told them that every word would be examined and criticized most minutely. . . . It is most difficult to stem the torrent of blind zeal." He expressed particular concern about Dubuisson's ardent effervescence and ended his note with the wry observation, "This miracle has caused a great deal of trouble—happy thing they do not occur often."[48]

The month of March was waning and Matthews began dreading the arrival of April, when Revs. Kohlmann and Dubuisson were to attempt a second series of cures in the city. But on April Fool's Day, he had new reason to worry. On that day, a scathing letter about the handling of the Mattingly miracle appeared in the *National Intelligencer* by a writer who used the pseudonym Democritus, after the ancient Greek philosopher known as the "laughing philosopher" because he advocated cheerfulness. Democritus began by declaring himself "a Catholic, but no enthusiast." He presented himself as an exemplar of the native camp, interested in blending Catholicism seamlessly into American culture.[49]

Ostensibly, Democritus wrote to correct an error in the *Baltimore Federal Gazette* that stated that Anthony Kohlmann was a Georgetown professor, when he was in fact superior at the Jesuit's White Marsh plantation. Democritus clearly wanted to distance Kohlmann from the college, and the attack seemed to have been motivated by strong personal antipathy. He proceeded to mock the pseudo-gothic story that had been published in newspapers in Philadelphia and New York about "'Father Confessor's spectacles and black cap,' and the 'beams of the moon' and the 'solitary casement,' and the 'breath of wind,' and the 'invisible hand.'" Writing in the well-established eighteenth-century genre of satire, he countered the elements of another popular eighteenth-century genre, the gothic.[50]

Democritus mercilessly skewered Kohlmann for his hyperbole in not explaining "how many [of the fifteen or sixteen witnesses] had to seek accommodation under the beds" in order to fit into the sickroom; for "having discovered that Mrs. Mattingly is the sister of her brothers, and the sister of her sisters"; and for his discovery of the answer to the "tough problem of finding the longitude" of Washington and Bamberg, which Democritus avers will save mariners' lives and earn him the reward of riding on the tail of a comet heading toward the sun. The letter ended with a call for information about other purported miracle attempts.[51]

Within a space of about three weeks after the miracle on March 10, the debate over the role of miracles in American Catholicism had begun in earnest. The two camps—Jesuit, or continental, enthusiast and Anglo-American, or native, moderate—were polarized. Contemporaries suspected that the author of Democritus's letter was Thomas C. Levins, who, like Democritus, was a mathematician and philosopher and who carried a grudge against Kohlmann for creating tensions at Georgetown College. With open disdain for the brand of enthusiastic piety of Kohlmann and Dubuisson, Levins mocked Jesuit rule books and said Mass only on Sundays—reportedly "at a 'gallop'" of only fifteen or sixteen minutes.[52] Levins had a taste for the scandalous poetry of Lord George Gordon Byron and others. His best friend was the English Jesuit Roger Baxter, a former literature professor at Georgetown who had left the college during the Kohlmann presidency. Because of their nonconformist views and scandalous behavior, their superior, Francis Dzierozynski, was, as early as February 1824, preparing to send the two back to Great Britain. By the time Democritus published his letter, Levins's friend Baxter had been reassigned to a remote mission in southern Maryland, and Levins was ostracized under a cloud of suspicion.

On April 5 a response from "A Catholic Layman," written the day after the publication of Democritus's letter, appeared in the *National Intelligencer,* doubting that Democritus could possibly be a Catholic. He stated that "the Catholics of Washington are universally indignant at his unmerited, unprovoked, and malignant attack upon a venerable and highly respected clergyman, for whom they entertain a warm affection and exalted esteem and regard." Although the writer could have been genuinely indignant about the attack on Kohlmann, it is likely that he was instead more uncomfortable with such a public airing of internal Catholic differences. The newspaper editor added this note, with the title, *Dr. Kohlmann's Letter,* "We have published the letter itself today and a brief note from one of his friends. *The National Journal* states, from authority, that 'the letter of Dr. Kohlmann was a private letter to a particular friend, expressing his individual opinion merely; that it was written in great haste, by no means intended for publication, and consequently, not for the purpose of provoking controversy.' Here, then, let the controversy end. The practice of publishing private letters of others, without their permission, leads to many unpleasant consequences." "A Catholic Layman" was trying to moderate Kohlmann's enthusiasm, by claiming his statements had not been prepared for publication, and to smooth the appearance of too many Catholic squabbles.[53]

Despite Layman's veiled plea for a cease-fire, the controversy continued. Democritus, deeply provoked, penned a scathing reply to the editors of the *National Intelligencer.* Had this been a speech, and "air quotes" invented, Democritus would have been their master, writing: "Gentlemen, works of supererogation should not remain unrecompensed. Allow me, then, to acknowledge the urbanity of 'Mr. Catholic Layman,' and to assure him and the 'Catholics of Washington, who are *universally* indignant,' that it is *not* 'pretty well ascertained' that Democritus is not a Catholic of this city. He *cannot* ascertain it . . . The 'attack' upon the letter was *not* malignant—it was *not* 'unmerited'—if Mr. 'Layman' could lay mental hold of a distinction, it was *not* 'unprovoked.'"[54] Democritus refused to back down, and underlying his concerns was the way Catholicism was being presented in light of the miracle. Whatever Washington's well-established Catholics thought about the controversies raging around the Mattingly cure is not known, but it had to be readily apparent to them that the continentalists and the natives had very different conceptions of what Catholicism should be in the United States.

Though his contemporaries and some Catholic historians today believe that Thomas C. Levins was both Democritus and Eberebron the Pilgrim, another pseudonym used by a writer criticizing the Mattingly miracle, he denied it. On April 7, 1824, he wrote to Roger Baxter: "It will spare me the trouble of forging one to express the excitement caused by a letter in the Intelligencer, which quizzed the production of the German. Whoever the wag was, he called himself Democritus; and not content with following in the steps of his ancient progenitor who only laughs per se at the follies of mankind—he has made others laugh and some *few* cry;—perhaps it wd be more proper to say, rain tears of vengeance and spite. You have already, probably, heard of this quiz Democritus from some of yr friends. If you have heard, it has also reached you that the *merits* of authorship have been donated to me. I need not say that they do not possess a shadow of proof against me—all rests on the most malignant suspicion."[55]

Levins goes on to tell how the "fanatical gang" have persecuted him under suspicion of the letter's authorship. This letter recounts that Jesuit superior Dzierozynski called a meeting of the Georgetown priests and demanded under their vow of obedience that they tell him whether any of them was indeed Democritus. Several of the priests said they were not, but Enoch Fenwick and Thomas Levins refused to answer the question. Levins stated to Baxter, "You prophesied correctly about the miracle—Kohlmann and the malicious Dubuisson, have nearly worked its ruin with their folly. . . . God help the poor miracle." He ends by sending Joseph Carbery, the priest and brother of Mrs. Mattingly, his best regards, and writes: "I trust he will not become on mere suspicion, an enemy. Suspicion, it appears, is enough for his brother the Captn."[56] Levins, then, was disavowing not the miracle, but its presentation to the world. For the Catholic clergy involved in debates over the miracle, very few of their differences had to do with faith and belief. They were far more concerned with how reception of the miracle would affect the developing American church.

A week later, Levins wrote directly to Joseph Carbery, nearly giddy with relief that Carbery had sent him a kind note and a ham. "You have heard of Democritus, and, that *suspicion* has identified me with that laughing gentleman," he wrote to Ann's brother. "Whoever he be, he has, to use an expression of the 'fancy,' sent Kohlmann to grass. This Dutchman has not had such a knock-down since he crossed the Atlantic." These are not exactly charitable sentiments, and in the same letter, he reveals that he expects Joseph Carbery to have read the letter he sent Baxter the week before, in which he also claimed he was not Democritus:

> I regret that yr brother Captn Carberry [*sic*] shd conceive that I could write anything bearing the interpretation of disrespect against his family. He floats upon the tide of genl suspicion— supposes me to be the author, and imagines that he is attacked, because the name of yr. sister, Mrs. Mattingly, is introduced. The fact is, Democritus says nothing of yr. sister but what is found in Kohlman's [*sic*] letter, and everyone, in the cool possession of his reflections, will acknowledge that his document only is the subject of remark. I did think that my character was sufficiently known to Captn Carberry, to believe that I am in-

capable of ever making the slightest allusion of disrespect to him
or his family. I trust you, at least, will not doubt my sincerity,
when I say that, *if I were Democritus, I could not be wanting in
decorum to your kindred* [italics added].[57]

The style of Levins's letters is florid and has similar sentence construction
to those of Democritus; it is in quite a different style than the writing of
Friend of Truth. In the letter to Joseph Carbery, he makes a point of saying
Democritus did not insult his sister, Ann Mattingly, and never fully denies
that he is the writer.

Following this sarcastic and contentious exchange in the Washington
press, Rev. Matthews was deeply concerned that a failure to have more cures
on April 10 would bring greater ridicule to the reports of the Mattingly
miracle, and he hoped to bring out a full report of the event before Congress
adjourned for the summer. Archbishop Maréchal anxiously awaited news of
how Congress responded to the sensational story. The English-born rector
of the Baltimore cathedral, James Whitfield, cautioned Maréchal against
repeating the mistake made by Daniel Murray, archbishop of Dublin, in
his encyclical on the cure of Mary Stuart—that of calling it "the effect of
a supernatural agency." Rev. Tessier himself wrote to Dubuisson that the
"Gentlemen of Baltimore," the archbishop and Whitfield, were having difficulty understanding the "zeal" over the miracle because they did not witness it. William Beschter also wrote that "everyone except Mr. Whitfield is
of the opinion that now he should give his pastoral letter."[58]

In fact, the archbishop's response was informed by a centuries-old de-
cree of the Council of Trent (1545–1563) that no new miracle shall be admitted without the recognition and approbation of a bishop. For centuries, the
Vatican had attempted to guard the church against overzealous immersion
into the supernatural by putting into place a process centered in rationality
and careful investigation. Maréchal had some of the same concerns about
the Washington miracle. He avoided sermonizing on it and did not issue an
encyclical. Maréchal's lukewarm enthusiasm for the miracle disappointed,
and even angered, the enthusiasts, whom Levins had dubbed "the friars."

Dubuisson wrote about his frustration in a letter to the archbishop, exclaiming, "It certainly behooves your grace to show great circumspection in pronouncing the cure to be a miracle, but it is my part to state the facts." Privately, the archbishop may have believed in the miracle, but he was very concerned about managing the public perception.[59]

In May 1824, the eagerly awaited *Collection of Affidavits and Certificates* was published with the approval of the archbishop and offered for sale at Guegan's bookstore in Washington. It contained twenty-seven affidavits and seven certificates. As the archbishop had advised, the witnesses, as he states himself, were well known for their "integrity, candour, and intelligence." Six prominent doctors gave testimony: William Jones, Alexander McWilliams, Nathaniel P. Causin, George A. Carroll, Thomas C. Scott, and James W. Roach. Mayor Carbery swore his affidavit in the presence of Chief Justice John Marshall of the U.S. Supreme Court. In addition to family members, other prominent Washingtonians attested to the cure: James Hoban, architect of the White House; Charles Sweeny, principal clerk of the Washington post office; circuit court judge Charles H. W. Wharton; and Harriet de la Palme Baker, wife of an American diplomat. This impressive list of important Washington citizens reflected the Sulpician ideal of public service and ecumenical cooperation and aligned more closely with the native camp.

During May, Anthony Kohlmann wrote to Peter Kenney about the tensions that boiled in Georgetown: "The College is as low as it can be, and cannot be continued but by a new set of men. The Archbp is sure to show his ill will to the Society [of Jesus] on every occasion—he has not and will never have the Whitmarsh [referring to the White Marsh plantation]. . . . There is open war at present, but unfortunately there is no union neither, and everything seems to be languishing." Kohlmann continued, writing about the reception of the miracle, "There has been an unaccountable apathy and indifference shown" and commented that Maréchal has forbid a pastoral letter.[60]

John England, bishop of Charleston, had been following with interest news of the cures of Prince Alexander Hohenlohe. His newspaper, the

Catholic Miscellany, had reprinted accounts of Barbara O'Connor's cure in England and of Mary Lalor and Mary Stuart in Ireland and had denounced a mean-spirited article that had been published in the *Edinburgh Review* during October 1823. While the printer's copyright on the *Collection of Affidavits* and the archbishop's prohibition prevented a reprinting of the documents in the *Catholic Miscellany,* Bishop England defended the reputation of Prince Hohenlohe. He refuted a statement that appeared in the *New York Evening Post* denying the possibility of contemporary miracles. On July 21, 1824, England published accounts of ten Hohenlohe cures that had reportedly occurred in France and the Netherlands.

Meanwhile, with the gradual return of her strength, Mrs. Mattingly resumed the duties of her former life. It was difficult, however, because she remained an object of intense interest to inquisitive strangers through the end of 1824 and beyond. Given nineteenth-century women's concerns about being covered prominently in the press, she was likely distressed over the negative attention that continued to appear during the rest of the year from such newspapers as the *National Journal,* the daily run by Thomas Carbery's political rival, Peter Force. Carbery had lost the mayoral election and was no longer in as prominent a role in the Federal City, so the critical articles in Force's newspaper likely had a double sting.

Six months after the cure, the controversy continued to be divisive. Thomas Levins became a target of another enthusiast, Brother Joseph Mobberly, who was at Georgetown College during October and November 1824. In his diary Mobberly wrote:

> Two or 3 days ago a piece appeared in one of the public papers ridiculing the miracle that was wrought last March in favour of Mrs Mattingly and ridiculing all those who believed it but especially those men in the City who for some time past have been styled Friars by way of ridicule. The Author seems to have written in the spirit of Democritus, who appeared against Revd Father Anth. Kohlman [*sic*] last march . . . The author is supposed not to be known and no doubt he supposes so himself,

but he is mistaken—Today at 1 O'clock, I heard him incautiously observe to his companion (who doubtless has a share in the business) that 'If we only could get _____ how we would tear these Friars to pieces.' His companions seemed alarmed gave him a prudential hint, & both walked off together to the other end of the porch, that they might be at a greater distance from the company. To the Author who has been so long scribbling his nonsense against the miracle good Father Kohlman & the virtuous catholics of Washington City has at length been discovered behind the post—And who would have thought it! A friend! A companion! A brother in office! A Brother in dignity! A brother in Jesus Christ! It has often been observed that the greatest enemies the Church ever had were her own Children.[61]

Though Mobberly is indignant that a Catholic would speak against the miracle, he is most alarmed that the publications continue.

Brother Mobberly congratulated himself on having identified the author who was now styling himself Eberebron the Pilgrim in the pages of the *National Journal*. Mobberly continued to write about the controversy during the month of November: "At dinner Revd T. Levins was suspended by the Rev. Fr. Sup. as being the author of the Pilgrims &c." He continues: "Last Saturday it was published in the Refectory that Rev. T. Levins having received his penance in silence & give edification was there absolved." Thomas Levins was ultimately dismissed from the Jesuit order by the superior, Aloysius Fortis.[62]

As much as Mobberly tried to counsel himself to forgive Levins, he could not, writing in his diary that Levins had a superior attitude toward others and believed "That man is a fool, this a goose & a 3d is a Jackass, & he [Levins] is the only wise man in existence!" The Mattingly miracle, then, had become a subject of intense fascination and a source of conflict. For enthusiasts such as Anthony Kohlmann, Stephen Dubuisson, and Joseph Mobberly, the American miracle was an event of great significance that would attract converts. Writing in November 1824 to Dubuisson of the cure, Dr. Peter Chotard of Baltimore observed that Ann Mattingly's "instantaneous and perfect cure is indeed a wonderful thing and I would betray my confreres were I to say that I do not see the finger of God in it."[63]

The moderates such as Rev. Matthews and the archbishop tried to steer their way through the shoals, grateful for Ann Mattingly's cure but leery of the precarious position in which it had placed the young American Catholic Church. In May 1824, Maréchal had written to a colleague in Quebec about the Mattingly miracle: "Everybody here believes that it was a miracle and even a very great miracle. Assuredly, this cure is very astonishing."[64] Moderating between the continental enthusiasts and the native Catholics in the Maryland tradition was a challenge for those in the middle. A few years later, the Irish-born John England would attempt to yoke a belief in modern miracles with a rational and evidence-based examination of the Mattingly cure.

The Body of Evidence

Historian and physician Jacalyn Duffin has identified several elements that are replayed in nearly every miraculous cure documented for the Vatican. First, the patient experiences an increase in suffering, which peaks during the months preceding the cure. Second, an invocation for a cure is made. Third, the healing occurs, followed, fourth, by the recognition of the event as a miracle. The fifth step is an expression of thanksgiving. All these elements are replicated in the Mattingly miracle. During the nearly seven-year period of her illness, Mrs. Mattingly's suffering increased, intensifying during the months before her cure. The invocation was the novena offered up by her friends. Her healing occurred, and it was recognized as a miracle. Expressions of gratitude followed. The steps of documenting the miracle were pursued by Bishop John England. He already had in hand a letter that Stephen Dubuisson had written him on March 11, 1824, that set out the agenda, "Say the incredulous what they will, *there* was *Digitus Dei*," the finger of God. Bishop England would agree with Dubuisson's assessment that "the God of nature will shew what his intentions were in granting so signal a benefit to our American church." England's strategy would be to champion the miracle by embracing the rationality and moderation of Rev. Matthews and Archbishop Maréchal with the quiet zeal of the enthusiasts like Dubuisson.[65]

Ann Carbery Mattingly would testify for both the 1824 and 1831 set of affidavits. She arose from her sickbed on March 10, 1824, and appeared before Justices of the Peace R. S. Briscoe and James Hoban two weeks after her cure on March 24. In her sworn statement, Mrs. Mattingly averred that several hundred people had visited her during those two weeks and that she considered God to be "the sole author of my restoration." She asserted that she had been on the verge of death and was now in good health. Thomas Carbery's affidavit details his sister's suffering in the days leading up to the cure that correspond with "occult cancer," as defined in eighteenth-century terminology: "The severity of the cancer had almost deprived her of the power to articulate—the left side and arm were very much contracted—her pulse was scarcely perceptible to the nicest touch—her tongue was hard, rough, and dark—her cough was the most incessant and distressing he ever heard, with chills, and her cheeks flushed with a hectic fever—her countenance greatly distorted with pain—she could not move herself in the bed, and had a constant spitting and puking of blood and fetid matter, that was almost insupportable." Two years later, in April 1826, he provided additional material that Bishop England requested regarding bedsores on Mrs. Mattingly's ulcerated back during her illness. Both pamphlets focus on a disturbing list of symptoms to demonstrate how miraculous was the cure.[66]

Her sisters, Ruth and Catharine, provided these details: "for about six months preceding their sister's sudden cure, she was afflicted with long, and apparently, very painful fits of hard arid dry coughing, and almost every fit was followed by a vomiting of blood, often mingled with corrupt and very offensive matter. That, during the space of about the last three weeks of her illness, she had daily chills and fevers, generally preceded by cold sweats and coldness of the extremities, and during the continuance of her chills, there was little or no intermission in her coughing." These severe symptoms are associated with late-stage breast cancer, but also with tuberculosis and mercury poisoning, which she may have developed because of her mercury treatments.[67]

Mrs. Mattingly's friend during the fourteen years she lived in Washington, Anne Maria Fitzgerald, stated, "Her sight was so much impaired at times, that she told me she could hardly recognize me; and for the few last days of her illness she complained of a constant noise in her head, resembling the tolling of bells, which affected her hearing very much." James Carbery added this:

> About three weeks before her restoration, violent chills regularly came on, about 4 o'clock in the afternoon of each day, and acting with the other symptoms greatly aggravated the disease. The vast quantities of feculent blood, which she cast up, led to the belief, that the whole interior of the stomach was ulcerated, if not in a state of mortification. It was often necessary to support her, sitting up in the bed, to prevent suffocation; and for this purpose, such was her debility, that it took two or three persons. Her appetite was entirely gone; taking nothing but laudanum to appease the pain, and small quantities of tea, (often administered from a tea spoon,) to abate a burning thirst. Frequently fainting from pain, and fatigue of coughing; and in this situation, she would remain a considerable time, without sensation or evincing any evidence of life, except a slight pulse. She was reduced to the very last extremity of life.

Lewis Carbery said:

> For the six months before her recovery, she has had an almost incessant cough, which, at times, was so protracted as to leave her in a state of complete apparent exhaustion, and so distressing to this deponent, that he has often been compelled to withdraw from her chamber—and that those fits were always accompanied and followed by puking large quantities of corrupted blood,

which often appeared to this deponent, to be strangling her,
and that this vomiting and spitting of blood, were her constant
attendants, through the whole six years of her confinement,
and so frequent has this unaccountable disease exhibited its
violence, that he cannot enumerate the number of times he has
been sent for to witness her death.

The graphic descriptions of the gruesome illness mark Mrs. Mattingly's
suffering as extraordinary; in her lack of complaint and offering up of her
suffering, she becomes the ideal symbol for Catholic womanhood, a "victim
soul."[68]

In the hours before the cure, five people were watching in Mrs. Mattingly's sickroom: Ruth Carbery, Catharine Carbery, Sybilla Carbery, Susan Mattingly, and Anne Maria Fitzgerald. Lewis Carbery came to witness
the taking of Communion, brought by Dubuisson. Mrs. Mattingly's brother
Thomas and her son John were called into the room after the sudden healing. Her pastor for nearly fourteen years, Rev. Matthews, testified that he
heard the news of her healing and hastened to see her. "When I arrived,
Mrs. Mattingly opened the door . . . [and] with a smiling countenance,
shook my hand," he testified. "Although prepared for this meeting, I could
not suppress my astonishment at the striking contrast produced in her person in a few hours; my mind had for years associated death, and her pale
emaciated face; a thrilling awe pervaded my whole frame."[69] Numerous
witness statements and testimonies that were collected would form the basis
of the first set of affidavits and of Bishop England's further investigation.

In England's subsequent report to Maréchal's successor, Rev. James
Whitfield, archbishop of Baltimore, who had given permission for England's multiyear investigation, England confessed his fascination with
the Mattingly cure, saying that he was most eager to "examine it specially."
England's desire to revisit the circumstances of the Mattingly miracle originated in a private visit that his sister Joanna England made with Ann Mattingly in 1826. During this interview, it was discovered that the "most pal-
pable evidence of the miraculous nature of the lady's cure, viz., the sudden

healing of an ulcerated back," had not been included in the initial reports of the miracle.[70] Not all of the details of the cure, then, had been previously known. England believed that many circumstances of the extraordinary case had been passed over, some through delicacy, and some in order not to overload the narrative with too many particulars, as it already contained so many facts. England, in keeping with Vatican protocol, wanted to prepare documents that would prove the existence of a modern miracle in the United States. Like all such official investigations, it had to rely on extensive evidence and documentation.

England's augmented narrative of forty-two pages, published in 1830 after six years of research, is extremely graphic in its descriptions. Throughout it, he includes vivid detail—often bringing in the testimony of multiple witnesses to corroborate a point over and over. Such details connect it strongly to the European tradition of miracles. The sufferings of Mrs. Mattingly and of others cured by Hohenlohe invoke the tradition of Catholic hagiography that argues for great suffering as a marker of great martyrdom. England's portrait of Mrs. Mattingly in agony recalls the torture instruments that pagans used against early church martyrs: at the height of her suffering, Mrs. Mattingly felt that she was being "bored with an auger, pinched with forceps, or cut with sharp instruments." This metaphorical language in the documents is blended with the scientific: "From the permanent contraction of the *pectoralis-major,* the left arm was kept applied to the side, and by its pressure greatly aggravated her sufferings. Constant pains were felt also under the scapula, and in the shoulder and arm of the left side." While the metaphorical language adds to the emotional power of the testimonies, the medical terminology adds to their credibility as evidence.[71]

England's documentation extensively delineates Mrs. Mattingly's sufferings. He details chest pain, internal burning, excessive thirst, and bedsores, writing, "I have been told myself by several respectable persons, that, for a considerable time, they found it extremely unpleasant and offensive to the smell to pass by her door." From the stench of her breath and diseased body, her doctors concluded that Mrs. Mattingly's cancer was "making rapid progress on the internal organs," and they "unhesitatingly declared that it would kill her." With the barest of pulse, and with the jaws of death yawning wide before her, Mrs. Mattingly lay immobile, waiting its approach.[72]

Through all these sufferings, the same witnesses averred, she "exercised a Christian fortitude, and practised a habitual piety and resignation, truly edifying and consolatory to her relatives and friends." In fact, because of her "extreme delicacy" and her wish to spare others the loathsome sight of the sores, Mrs. Mattingly would lie in bed fully dressed. During the final days of her illness, with her sight failing, she suffered from a "constant noise in her head, resembling the tolling of bells," and requested her attendants "to bathe her head with vinegar, as she said she felt a violent pain in it." Additional pains in her side and breast convinced the patient that "mortification had taken place" and death was very near. All witnesses corroborate the evidence that Mrs. Mattingly's body was, as her brother termed it, "a wreck of sickness and corruption." Her body, in its most decayed state, would be a perfect metaphor for what Jenny Franchot has termed Protestant America's association of Catholics with "disease, death, and decomposition." For Protestants of this period, Catholicism seemed unhealthily connected to a deviant corporeality. Franchot develops this contrast, which seems appropriate for such compilations of symptoms: "If the symbolic terrain of Protestantism figured itself as clean, empty, and magically capable of change without delay, that of Catholicism was clogged with the filth of bodies."[73]

Even as he compiled the extensive, repetitive details of Mrs. Mattingly's agonizing illness, England cautioned readers who might respond squeamishly to these written descriptions that the actual sufferings and cure were far more compelling:

> I have found on this as on several other occasions, how much more satisfactory and distinct the testimony is which one derives from *viva voce* examination, than from any written documents. I shall never forget the description to me of the occurrences of that morning! . . . The tumour had disappeared; the ulcers on

her back had healed, without leaving a vestige (not even a cica-
trix) of their late ravages. Her breath, lately so intolerably fetid
and disgusting, was become very pleasant; and a sweet taste
substituted for the very disagreeable one which had so long
existed in her mouth. She could now use her left arm as well
as ever; and could throw it into any posture she chose, without
occasioning the slightest pain.[74]

England's focus in gathering this evidence was to provide incontro-
vertible proof that the miracle had occurred. In 1828, Rev. Stephen Dubuisson prepared an extraordinary letter to Bishop England with additional
details of Mrs. Mattingly's illness. Because of "delicacy of feeling," he said,
Mrs. Mattingly had not mentioned the constipation of her bowels from
which she suffered before her cure. Following the restoration of her health,
an "easy natural movement took place." From this intensely intimate bodily
detail, Dubuisson then moves to a discussion that almost suggests he was
considering putting Mrs. Mattingly forth as a candidate for sainthood. He
writes that Mrs. Mattingly informed him that "as often as she approaches
the holy table, she continues to experience the same physical and delicious
flavor . . . [that] has frequently left in her mouth a delightsome fragrance
with which her face, hands, and veil are frequently perfumed."[75]

England, through his accumulation of original and additional evidence, was satisfied that a splendid miracle had occurred. To Archbishop
Whitfield, he confidently stated, "Such a body of witnesses has seldom
been arrayed for the purpose of satisfying the public mind . . . I unhesitatingly assert, that a more respectable aggregate of witnesses, to any series
of facts, never came under my observation." But Bishop England's newly
published documentation of the miracle in 1830, though scientific and rational, did not finally fulfill his hope to elevate the Catholic Church in the
United States. The unflinching descriptions of bodily illness in England's
collection probably would have both attracted and repelled Catholic and
Protestant readers. In January 1830, the newspaper the *Protestant* was
launched with the avowed purpose of warning the nation of the dangers of

Popery. Anti-Popery had been revived in the United States, the beginnings of what Ray Allen Billington has called the Protestant Crusade. By the 1830s, such dwelling on the female body played into Protestant suspicions about priests and nuns in Catholic monasteries and fueled the rising threat of anti-Catholic violence that would erupt during the next two decades.[76]

SIX

Aftermath

What, I say, is miracle, what is magic, what are the dreams of miracle,
the superstitions of magic, in comparison with the results of plain work
which God puts in our power? Ask a miracle of God,—and there is
no answer. The world is the answer, and it lies before us.

—Theodore Parker, *Lessons from the World of Matter
and the World of Man* (1865)

Washington, D.C., 1844

Sailors are a notoriously superstitious lot. Once a tragedy happens aboard a
ship, savvy sailors typically steer clear of the unlucky vessel, and the boat,
no matter how magnificent, can be idled for lack of a crew. Such was the
case with a seemingly cursed American ship, the USS *Princeton,* which was
built for war and launched on September 5, 1843. Though not larger than a
typical nineteenth-century warship, 164 feet long and a little more than 30
feet wide, it was the most technologically advanced vessel of its day, with
an iron hull. Designed by a Swedish engineer, John Ericsson, who would
became famous two decades later for his Civil War battleship the *Monitor,*
the steamship *Princeton* was equipped with three masts, a full suit of sails,
and a thin telescopic smokestack. It moved swiftly through the water, sails
furled, even during a dead calm, thanks to its remarkable seawater-cooled
engine that lay deep in the hull, ten feet below the waterline. The coal-
burning engine, invulnerable to attack through the iron hull, was so clean
and efficient that no smoke was visible coming from the ship even at top
speed. Anyone who watched the *Princeton* slide through the water on a
windless day, as if by magic rather than by steam, would understand why
some called it the "Phantom Ship."

On an unusually temperate last day of February 1844, a crowd of elite Washingtonians gathered for an excursion down the Potomac on the *Princeton*. The steam sloop's charismatic captain, Robert F. Stockton, described as "a man whose appearance more favorably impresses you with his qualifications as a man and a sailor," had invited scores of journalists, members of Congress and the cabinet, and President John Tyler—altogether more than three hundred guests—on board for a day trip. President Tyler's fiancée, Julia Gardiner; her sister; and the president's father-in-law-to-be, former New York State senator David Gardiner, were special guests. Dolley Madison was aboard. So was most of the cabinet, including Abel P. Upshur, recently elevated to secretary of state; the new secretary of the navy, Thomas W. Gilmer; and Virgil Maxcy, a lawyer and former member of the Maryland State Senate. From the Senate and House came Thomas Hart Benton, John C. Calhoun, and a score of others "to feast their eyes on this nautical wonder, this gem of the ocean, this last effort of American genius, skill, and architectural ingenuity."[1]

As the historian Donald B. Webster Jr. also noted, the *Princeton* was "perhaps the most powerful warship the world had ever seen," both a "national status symbol" and "visible evidence of the nation's growing naval power and ambition." Among other marvels, it featured the largest cannon ever mounted on a ship. The Peacemaker, as it was called, was fourteen feet long and weighed twenty-five thousand pounds; in a dramatic demonstration on the trip out, it had fired a cannonball four miles. Over an elegant lunch of pheasant and ham, Stockton served his guests copious amounts of champagne, sherry, and brandy and boasted that the cannon could clear the British out of contested Oregon.[2]

On the return trip, Secretary of the Navy Gilmer requested that the Peacemaker be fired again. While most of the guests, including President Tyler, continued their revels in the main cabin, a small number assembled on deck to watch another demonstration of the monstrous cannon. This group included Secretary Upshur, Senator Benton, David Gardiner, Virgil Maxcy, and a handful of others. The gun crew loaded the Peacemaker with a light charge, twenty-five pounds of powder, and Stockton took a position to fire the piece himself. Webster tells what happened next:

Stockton pulled the lanyard to trigger the gun's lock, and the whole ship shook with the force of a great explosion; even the revelers in the main cabin felt it. A thick cloud of white smoke rolled over the vessel, and from it came a few low moans, nothing else. As the smoke cleared, a scene almost beyond comprehension greeted the eyes of the onlookers: The Peacemaker had burst apart along its left side, shattering into flying fragments several thousand pounds of iron from the mounting trunnions backward. Stockton lay on the deck, luckily only stunned, with a big piece of metal lying on his chest. Two sailors lifted it away and hauled their bloody and shaken captain erect. He surveyed the terrific carnage at his feet.

The Secretary of the Navy was dead; a piece of metal had evidently killed him instantly and then gone on to hit Secretary of State Upshur, who had been standing directly behind him. Upshur, struck in the head, died before medical aid could reach him. Mrs. Gilmer, who throughout the day had never lost her feeling of foreboding, was miraculously unhurt, but now gave way to uncontrollable hysterics. Along with Gilmer and Upshur, everyone standing to the left of the Peacemaker had been literally mowed down by the hail of shattered iron. Virgil Maxcy had lost both arms and a leg and died instantly. David Gardiner and Commodore Beverly Kennon, Chief of the Navy's Bureau of Construction, lay unconscious, mortally wounded. The ship's surgeons could do nothing for either of them.

Senator Benton, seated on another gun about six feet away from the Peacemaker, saw the cannon fire, felt a blast in the face, and knew nothing more until he woke up, suffering from shock and a burst ear drum, a few minutes later. President Tyler's personal servant of many years had been standing next to Benton. He was dead, as were two sailors in the gun crew. Nine others were wounded, some critically.[3]

A writer in the *National Intelligencer* mused on the meaning of the tragedy: "in this catastrophe . . . there is an obvious rebuke of that spirit of vaunting confidence which certainly forms a shade in our character as a people! That arm which has both uplifted and thus far upheld us, but which we are all too prone to forget, terribly and signally smote us . . . in the very act and hour of our high exultation."[4] A chastened nation contemplated the hubris of Promethean overreaching. This powerful force smiting several victims at once is, of course, the antithesis of the healing touch of a miracle, but both can be read as powerful supernatural messages.

After state funerals for the victims, the *Princeton* was repaired, and Captain Stockton was exonerated, the investigating committee finding that explosions on ships were part of the risk of sailing on them. The *Princeton* served briefly in the Mexican War under another skipper, then Stockton took it on a grand tour of Europe, where government officials and huge crowds greeted it in every port with the same adulation it had received in the United States five years earlier. At home, though, the *Princeton* never regained the sparkling and ghostly presence that had awed public and government alike. It was, in fact, considered a jinxed ship by the Navy Department, which was still wary of innovations and distrustful of the *Princeton* in particular. Once Stockton retired from the navy and successfully ran for Congress, the Phantom Ship was decommissioned, broken apart, and scrapped.

The Mattingly family apparently had a connection to one of the victims on the *Princeton,* the former senator from Maryland, Virgil Maxcy. Thomas Joseph Mattingly, Ann Mattingly's grandson, and his wife Hannah Reeves named their firstborn son Virgil Maxcy Mattingly. The specific connection between the Mattinglys and Maxcy is, however, unknown. The baby was born September 23, 1854, ten years after the *Princeton* explosion. Within six months, his great-grandmother, Ann Mattingly, would die at age seventy. It is doubtful that Ann ever saw her newborn great-grandson Virgil because at the time of his birth, his father, Thomas Joseph, was outcast from the family, as was his sister, Annie Elizabeth Mattingly. Neither of these two children of Ann's son John Baptist Carbery Mattingly nor any of their children were named as heirs in Ann's will—or in any Carbery wills,

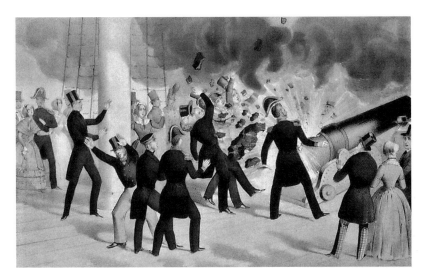

Explosion on the USS *Princeton* from a print by Currier and Ives. Courtesy of the Library of Congress.

for that matter. After her miraculous cure, Ann developed a permanent estrangement from her son, John, and all his descendents. Little Virgil Maxcy Mattingly died about two months before his fifth birthday on July 8, 1859. No information is given about this tragedy, and the only notation on his burial record from Glenwood Cemetery is that the child was "white."[5]

Ann Mattingly's Body

Just as with little Virgil Maxcy Mattingly, there is much we do not know about his great-grandmother, Ann Carbery Mattingly. No photographs of her have surfaced, and no diaries have been found. The documents that remain are few: a handful of letters and affidavits relating to her cure, and her last will and testament. A small box of relics, religious and devotional items belonging to her, is in the collection of the Georgetown Visitation Monastery. Of the seven decades of her life, she lived only one in relative celebrity. And after that celebrity, Mrs. Mattingly seems to have withdrawn

Rosary beads
belonging to Ann
Mattingly. Photo
by John Holloway.
Collection of
Georgetown
Visitation
Monastery
Archives.

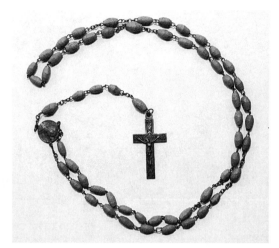

into privacy during the last twenty years of her life, living with her daughter, son-in-law, and their children and denied her deepest wish to live out the remainder of her life in the seclusion of a convent. But for a woman so unknown in conventional ways, we know a great deal about her body. As we have seen, the trials of her illness were exhaustively documented. Thus, we know things about Ann Mattingly that we will never learn about, for instance, George Washington or John Adams: the color of her stool during her illness, the texture of her vomit, and the stench of her breath. We know this much, in part, because of the key role gender explicitly and implicitly played in the response to the miracle of her cure in 1824.

Mrs. Mattingly is not the typical heroine found in books. She was a deeply religious woman, given much more to meditation and contemplation than her brief celebrity as the beneficiary of two miracles might suggest. Part of her personality was certainly shaped by her girlhood in southern Maryland, where she imbibed the culture of Catholicism. Part of that culture, and an essential difference between Protestantism and Catholicism, lies in the perception of the body, with Catholicism largely perceived as a more "feminized" religion. Within these gendered associations of "muscular" Protestantism and feminized Roman Catholicism, the doctrine of tran-

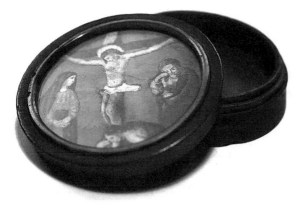

Rosary bead box belonging to Ann Mattingly. Photo by John Holloway. Collection of Georgetown Visitation Monastery Archives.

substantiation offers the most dramatic contrast between the two versions of Christianity. For Protestants, the bread and wine blessed upon the altar *represent* the body and blood of Christ; for Catholics, they *are* the body and blood of Christ. In a sense, even Catholicism's sacrament of confession, focused on the salvation of the soul, takes on a kind of physicality in that the male priest has the power to free the soul of the stain of sin at the moment of absolution. As the scholars Ann Taves and Marie Pagliarini have shown, the doctrine of the real presence and the "eucharocentric" devotions it encouraged were central to the foundations of American Catholic devotional practice in the nineteenth century. The mediation of the Eucharist also enhanced the stature of the priest's role in church ritual, as he functions as the instrument for the miracle of transubstantiation.[6]

This physicality of the sacraments is intimately linked to Prince Alexander Hohenlohe's miraculous cures; in fact, both transubstantiation and confession are invoked in the prayer penned by Hohenlohe and translated by Rev. Dubuisson, "Oh God . . . let thy power and majesty shine on account of thy servant *in the same manner as thou actest in the consecration by the words of the Priest, in changing the bread and wine into the true Body and Blood of Jesus Christ, and in the same manner thou doest by thy immediate power, in the words of absolution* . . . with firm belief and confidence that thou willst act in an immediate manner, I in the Name of Jesus Christ commend by the power given me in holy Baptism,—these infirmities to remove" (italics added). The healing of the body is inextricably linked to the healing of the soul. Both transubstantiation and miraculous cures, then, were performed by male clergy and documented by male physicians. Bishop John England sent the affidavits from his subsequent investigation of Mrs. Mattingly's cure to a group of eminent physicians at the South Carolina Medical Society in Charleston and at the prestigious medical college there, but they never issued a position statement.[7]

Nineteenth-century Catholicism, with its emphasis on the separation of realms of experience, or spheres, of men and women, fostered what Barbara Welter has called "the cult of true womanhood," enacted in the female virtues of piety, purity, submission, and domesticity. More recently, historian Paula Kane has observed, "Perhaps no topic in the study of the history of religion provokes more debate than that of gender." Kane offers a definition of *gender* in contrast to *sex* as a social construction that "implies a system of rules, ideologies, and institutions that define, regulate, and enforce what it means to be a man and a woman." Any complete interpretation of the controversies surrounding the Mattingly miracle and the aftereffects on family relations must build on an analysis of nineteenth-century conceptions of masculinity and femininity, and an understanding of how women's bodies were considered during this period.[8]

Certainly, the diagnosis of Ann Mattingly's illness was filtered through the prism of gender. As was typical with nineteenth-century female invalids, her male physicians partially attributed her maladies to gynecological problems. One attending doctor, as John England's investigative documents note, "believed that the haemorrhage was vicarious; nor did he abandon this opinion until convinced by Mrs. M. that the functions of her uterus (except when she was very much reduced) continued to be performed." Her doctor, in other words, believed that that offensive blood Mrs. Mattingly was vomiting in 1824 was the function of menstruation. In the specialized language of physiology, the word *vicarious* means that one organ is performing functions normally performed by another. In Mrs. Mattingly's case, then, the physician believed that the vomit, which one witness described as "so clotted as to appear like liver" and another as "a mixture of matter resembling pieces of flesh," was in fact the rerouted monthly flow of Mrs. Mattingly's menstrual period.[9]

This publication of what Marie Pagliarini calls "very personal and seemingly inappropriate information" puts the framers of the cure narratives on a par with God's "all-seeing gaze." Furthermore, the significant role of gender in the reception of the Mattingly miracle is demonstrated by Friend of Truth's casting doubt on the seriousness of Mrs. Mattingly's illness. After discussing her symptoms with "five medical men," Friend of Truth charged that Mrs. Mattingly's illness was not cancer at all, but an abscess that broke. The opinions of the doctors, all male of course, are in marked contrast to the affidavits of the "five Roman Catholic ladies" whom Friend so summarily dismissed in his refutation. When Eberebron the Pilgrim wrote in the pages of the *National Journal* that supporters of the Mattingly miracle were "petulant & snarling old women," he exposed the depth of the role of gender in this story. Rev. Joseph Clorivière delivered a sermon on April 19, 1824, in the midst of the battles over the Mattingly miracle, in which he stated: "But Our Lord has chosen the weak things of this world to confound the great—Women in general have more susceptibility of heart—less pride of mind—& without here meaning or willing it be thought that I compliment them in this place—Our Lord made them the 1st instruments of his grace. . . . I know not why the opinion and testimony of women should not be believed in matters of religion—which require more purity of heart than science." His seemingly inadvertent condescension may be just a slight improvement over the blatant misogyny of the period.[10]

The language used in the 1830s to allege depravity toward women "imprisoned" in convents is grounded in earlier discussions of Roman Catholic miracles. But what is there in the cure of illness that these Protestant detractors found filthy, obscene, and grossly immoral? Widespread in the documents connected to the cures are frank and graphic descriptions of the female body. Nineteenth-century readers critical of Catholicism certainly would have responded negatively to these unflinching details, which are shocking even today.

After the miracle of 1824, others appropriated Mrs. Mattingly's body for their own purposes, breaking the usual taboos of privacy and intimacy. As Pagliarini has noted about Catholic miraculées, including Ann Mattingly, their bodies were viewed as signs "that bore the traces of spiritual truth," and these messages were decoded and interpreted. "Those authorized to read women's bodies were male," says Pagliarini, "and they were generally either doctors or members of the Catholic hierarchy." Typically, biographies are chronological and based on events—most often, dramatic events that are outwardly enacted. Ann Mattingly's biography is a series of shards and fragments—because the events of her life did not seem to others as valuable to document as her miraculous cure. But Mrs. Mattingly may have one of the most well-documented bodies of any woman in the nineteenth century—along with Fanny Burney, another a breast cancer survivor who penned in 1812 a harrowing description of her mastectomy without anesthesia. The conflicts over the meaning of the miracle reveal important attitudes about gender in the early national period.[11]

Furthermore, Ann Mattingly's disease, breast cancer, carries with it many burdensome metaphors, so brilliantly articulated by Susan Sontag in her 1978 essay "Illness as Metaphor." Sontag, while herself in treatment for cancer, dissected the notion of the "cancer personality" and confronted the way that the universal terror of this disease has turned it into a powerful metaphor, a metaphor that does great harm to cancer patients. In her essay, Sontag unpacks what she calls the *obscenity* of cancer, true to the etymology of the word *obscene:* "ill-omened, abominable, repugnant to the senses." Sontag reviews early definitions of cancer in the Oxford English Dictionary, "Anything that frets, corrodes, corrupts, or consumes slowly and secretly." The word itself comes from the Greek *karkínos* and the Latin *cancer,* which means crab—inspired by the resemblance of the swollen veins in an external tumor to a crab's legs. Sontag is primarily interested in the concept of illness as metaphor, but it is important to understand that a gendered conception of cancer underlies both Sontag's discussion and responses to Ann Mattingly's primarily "female" disease.[12]

One of the most damaging pieces of the cancer metaphor is the notion of the "cancer personality." While tuberculosis (which, for instance, killed the poet John Keats in 1820) was romanticized in the nineteenth century as a disease resulting from too much passion and sensuality, Sontag observes, "cancer is a disease of insufficient passion, afflicting those who are sexually repressed, inhibited, unspontaneous, incapable of expressing anger." Sontag notes that psychiatrist Wilhelm Reich defined cancer as "a disease following emotional resignation—a bio-energetic shrinking, a giving up of hope." Reich, writing in the twentieth century, would have found ample evidence in Ann Mattingly's failed marriage to suggest that such emotional resignation and shrinking of hope would not be surprising.[13]

This lingering view of the cancer personality is rooted in medical documents dating from the late eighteenth century that are implicitly gendered in their conception. In 1759, Richard Guy, a surgeon, wrote of Ann Mattingly's diagnosis, a "scirrhus" in the breast, that it was "not uncommon to married or unmarried, young or middle-aged Women, especially those who are subject to Hysteric and nervous complaints . . . but seem peculiar to certain constitutions as the dull, heavy, phlegmatic, and melancholic." Tumors of the type found in Ann Mattingly's breast were also described in a widely read eighteenth-century textbook by William Buchan as "a hard indolent tumour seated in some of the glands; as the breasts, the armpits, &c." Its cause was thought to originate in "suppressed evacuations of old maids and widows, about the time when the menstrual flux ceases." Buchan elaborated further on these additional causes: "It may likewise be occasioned by excessive fear, grief, anger, religious melancholy, or any of the depressing passions. Hence the unfortunate, the choleric, and those persons who devote themselves to a religious life in convents or monasteries, are often afflicted with it." We have previously noted that in Mrs. Mattingly's era, breast cancer was known as the "nun's disease."[14]

The descriptions of Ann Mattingly's advanced illness echo the descriptions found in Buchan's text of "occult cancer," which, he writes, "seems often very trifling at the beginning . . . a hard tumor about the size of a hazel nut, or perhaps smaller, is generally the first symptom . . . The pain and stench become unbearable; the appetite fails; the strength is

Relic box owned
by Mary Susan
Mattingly Lay,
Ann Mattingly's
daughter.
Photo by John
Holloway.
Collection of
Georgetown
Visitation
Monastery
Archives.

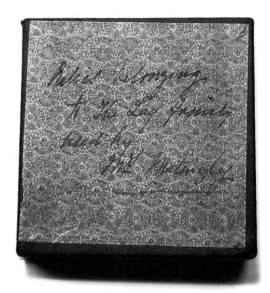

exhausted by a continual hectic fever; at last, a violent hemorrhage, or discharge of blood, from some part of the body; with faintings, or convulsion
fits, generally puts an end to the miserable patient's life." The descriptions
of Mrs. Mattingly's illness by numerous witnesses appear to corroborate
the diagnosis of advanced breast cancer.[15]

Ann Mattingly was a widow by age thirty-eight. By the time of her
husband's death in 1822, she was confined to bed, and we know from asides
in some of the sworn affidavits about the cure that she did not attend his
funeral. She certainly suffered from grief, and possibly anger, at the circumstances of her life. She was estranged from her husband, with no recourse to
divorce because of her social standing and religion. She worried about her
children, especially her son John, as illustrated by her poignant deathbed
plea to her aunt Carbery and her pastor William Matthews to love them
once she was gone. Her mother, her sister-in-law, a beloved uncle, and her
husband had died during her seven-year illness.

She was deeply religious, and after her cure, she wished to devote
herself to religious life at the Georgetown Visitation Monastery, but this

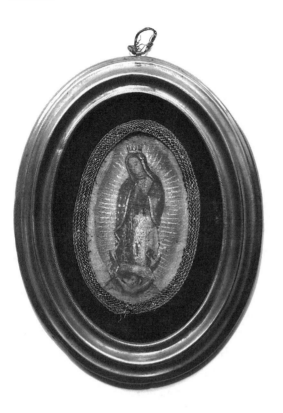

Miniature of the Blessed Virgin Mary belonging to Ann Mattingly. Photo by John Holloway. Collection of Georgetown Visitation Monastery Archives.

wish remained unfulfilled at her death in 1855. Among the relics in her family's possession after she died were a portrait of Prince Hohenlohe, an image of the Blessed Virgin, rosary beads, and a crucifix. Ann Mattingly also owned a "discipline," a small whip or scourge, used for self-inflicted mortification. The practice of such an austerity is most typically carried out under the guidance of a spiritual advisor. According to *A Catholic Dictionary*, mortification may be "practised for the motive of expiation of past sins, whether of oneself or of others." It is not known whether Ann Mattingly mortified the flesh of her healed body, either for her own sins or those of, perhaps, her husband and son. That it was found among her possessions is suggestive. Mrs. Mattingly's body, like the bodies of many antebellum women, was almost always under the control of men. But with the self-cure of her foot in 1831, and perhaps with her spiritual discipline, Ann Mattingly may have been trying to wrest a larger degree of control over it.[16]

Mrs. Mattingly's miraculous cure literally embodied tensions in American culture between the religious and the secular that were forged at the nation's founding in the decreed separation of church and state. Her healing in 1824 took place at the intersection of religion and medicine, an apt microcosm of dialectic between faith and reason that animated the early republican era during which she lived. The cure made visible what was typically unseen in early American culture. Mrs. Mattingly's diseased body became a central object at the junction of mind and spirit during a period when a social order for the nation was being built. For ultimately, the process of answering the body's needs and desires is what creates a nation's language, culture, social institutions, and laws. Mrs. Mattingly's illness and cure subliminally reminded those at work building the Capital City and the nation that society is a corporation of individual bodies. In the nation's capital, then—with the word *capital* itself deriving from the bodily metaphor of *the head*—the widow's experiences underscored that the mind and body of the new republic are codependent—and that the primitive lurks just under the veneer of the civilized. The prominent role of a woman's body, first enslaved to a devastating illness and then miraculously emancipated by the hand of God, raised an uncomfortable specter in the emerging debates over the roles of both women and slaves in the new republic.[17]

Slavery, Race, and the Mattingly Miracle

In addition to internal conflicts within the Catholic Church and the role of gender, slavery was another significant feature of the historical context for the Mattingly miracle. We know that the Carberys owned slaves in Washington, one of whom, "old Hanna," helped care for Ann Mattingly and lived to be one hundred years old. John England, who played such an important role in investigating the miracle, was, despite his personal reservations, a public apologist for slavery. In essence, the Catholic Church shrank away from the condemnation of slavery by labeling it a political issue best left to

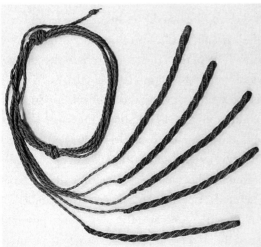

"Discipline" (two views) owned by Ann Mattingly. Photos by John Holloway. Collection of Georgetown Visitation Monastery Archives.

the legislature to solve. For this position, Catholic leaders found support in their theology, which stressed personal salvation through the sacraments and disengagement from social reform. Nineteenth-century church leaders, then, did not readily don the cloak of moral responsibility for slavery in the United States.[18]

The Jesuits, who play such a large role in the Mattingly controversy, had a long history of owning and using slaves on their Maryland plantations, and these slaves must be considered an integral part of the property disputes referred to in Chapter 5. Members of the Society of Jesus had arrived in the American colonies with the plan of using revenues from their estates to support their mission to the settlers and Indians, having been granted several thousand acres in original charters from Lord Baltimore in 1636. Andrew White, the first Jesuit in Maryland, brought two mixed-race serving men with him during 1633–1635, but these were probably indentured servants, not slaves. The Jesuits had, in fact, planned to use indentured servants to work their estates, but this kind of labor quickly became scarce in the new nation. So like their secular counterparts in Maryland, the Jesuits turned to slave labor. Historian R. Emmett Curran writes: "Although there is explicit evidence of Jesuit slaves only from 1711 on, it is highly probable that they were working on plantations for at least a generation by that time. By 1765 there were 192 such slaves."[19]

When Pope Clement XIV suppressed the Jesuits in 1773, members of the order living in colonial Maryland, unlike Jesuits in other nations, were able to keep their properties. The Maryland Jesuits were in this unique position because there was as yet no bishop in the colonies to seize the properties; the nearest bishop was in Quebec and had little jurisdiction over Maryland lying seven hundred miles to the south. In order to legally regulate their holdings, the Jesuits chartered themselves in 1783 as the Select Body of the Clergy, then in 1792 as the Corporation of Roman Catholic Clergymen. John Carroll, who had been named bishop of Baltimore, became the director, and, by law, only American citizens could be members of the Select Body. With this charter, the American trustees were empowered to administer the property of the suppressed Jesuits, distribute revenue, approve expenditures, and oversee the general business of the estates. The predominantly foreign superiors of the order, then, had no legal authority over the property of American Jesuit missions. Even once the Society of Jesus was reestablished in 1805, the corporation remained separate, providing a practical distinction between the temporal and spiritual realms. The corporation retained its former estates and possessions, including its slaves.[20]

Curran has demonstrated that this arrangement resulted in "persistent tensions" between the native Jesuits and their continental brethren. European superiors, such as Giovanni Antonio Grassi and Anthony Kohlmann, a key participant in the Mattingly miracle, were viewed as "ignorant monarchists" incapable of understanding American republicanism and the unique role of the corporation as a large Maryland landowner. The continental superiors were resented by their American counterparts for incurring large debts to finance educational projects such as Georgetown College and the Washington Catholic Seminary and for admitting large numbers of European novices, who then needed financial support. Francis Dzierozynski, from Russia, and Stephen Dubuisson, who had left Santo Domingo with his parents during the revolution there, according to Curran, "found the American Jesuits too independent, too materialistic, and too little observant of the rules of religious life." And the European superiors, for their part, blamed bad management of the estates for the nearly $32,000 debt of the Jesuit mission by 1822. Arguments over slaves and other property, then, divided along the same lines as divisions over the Mattingly miracle.[21]

The practice of Catholic priests participating in the "peculiar institution" was controversial. Debates heated up over the disposition of slaves on their plantations and especially over the question of whether or not priests should own slaves. As early as the fall of 1814, the Corporation of Roman Catholic Clergymen had begun considering a plan to free its slaves. John Carroll wrote in 1815, "since the great stir raised in Engld. about Slavery, my Brethren being anxious to suppress censure, which some are always glad to affix to the priesthood, have begun some years ago, and gradually proceeding to emancipate the old population on their estates." By 1820, the plan had been abandoned. Curran attributes the change of heart over emancipation in part to the appointment of Ambrose Maréchal as archbishop of Baltimore as successor to Carroll.[22]

We have seen in Chapter 5 that Maréchal initiated claims against the Jesuit estates such as White Marsh on the grounds that they were meant to support the church in Maryland, not merely the Jesuits. The disputed claim may have delayed the planned mass sale of slaves. Significantly, Maréchal chose to make his claim not in the U.S. courts, but in Rome. In July 1823, when Pope Pius VII ordered the Maryland Jesuits to surrender the White Marsh plantation with all its slaves and equipment to the archbishop, the Jesuits defied the order, claiming that their charter as a corporation rendered this a civil matter—an area, therefore, in which a bishop had no rights. Even after the miracle, in May 1824, Kohlmann was vowing to never surrender White Marsh to Maréchal. In the months immediately before and after the U.S. government's declaration of the Monroe Doctrine, the internal battles over both the miracle and slavery within the American Catholic Church took on intense significance.[23]

On March 25, 1824, just fifteen days after Ann Mattingly was cured, Aloysius Fortis, a Jesuit General in Rome, had written to Francis Dzierozynski, an active promoter of the miracle, urging him to break the power of the corporation as an independent authority. His letter revealed the disgust of the so-called European friars at the Maryland Jesuits' attachment to secular property: "Let them renounce the property, and God will bless their work," he wrote. The Jesuits countered that if Rome seized White Marsh, it would constitute foreign interference with the civil rights of U.S. citizens. On October 24, 1824, just months after the Mattingly cure, George Brent, the chief clerk of the Department of State, warned the archbishop that "the government of the United States . . . can never view with indifference any future appeals to such foreign states, touching the administration of temporal concerns under its jurisdiction." As time passed, some foreign-born Jesuits, such as Anthony Kohlmann and Stephen Dubuisson, gained admission to the corporation, and the Maryland Jesuits brought the administration of the property under the control of the superior or provincial.[24]

Brother Mobberly, who managed St. Inigoes parish from 1806 to 1820 and excoriated Rev. Thomas C. Levins for his treachery with regard to the Mattingly miracle, seems to have experienced the hardening of heart that Harriet Beecher Stowe, in *Uncle Tom's Cabin,* warned was the fate of overseers, writing in his diary, "the better a Negro is treated, the worse he becomes." The Jesuits' thin resources had to be stretched to support both the plantations and the fledgling educational project at Georgetown. With the economic downturn of the early 1820s, the living conditions for slaves of the Jesuit plantation grew much worse. By 1823, even the novices on the White Marsh plantation were subsisting on bread and water. That year, Father McSherry, assistant to the Georgetown president, began to sell the slaves to meet financial needs; between 1823 and 1843, the Jesuits sold slaves to pay off the debts of Georgetown College and other debts of the corporation. In 1831, the Jesuit superior general estimated that Jesuits still owned four hundred slaves, which made the order one of the nation's largest slaveholders. In 1838, facing financial difficulties, it sold some of its slaves, and in 1843, the sale of all remaining slaves from the four estates in southern Maryland raised $115,000, the equivalent of nearly $3.5 million today.[25]

Ann Mattingly's brother, Rev. Joseph Carbery, was one of a few priests who managed to improve the financial condition of the plantations, as well as the lives of the slaves, by the 1830s. At St. Inigoes, Carbery demonstrated the family business acumen by dividing the estate into seven farms. One farm was rented to a white farmer, and five others were assigned to slave families at an annual charge of $1.25 per acre. The families were responsible for providing for all their own needs, a free enterprise experiment that resulted in incentives for the slaves to produce for their own profit. Carbery worked the seventh farm himself, with the help of approximately half of the active slaves. By this period, many of the Jesuit slaves were able to earn about $100 per year by doing extra work for their owners, or by selling commodities they had grown, made, or caught. The developing battle over slavery within the early Catholic Church in the United States was an important undercurrent in the response to the Mattingly miracle. The question of race would also directly touch the Mattingly and Carbery families.[26]

Nemini Cedimus: John Baptist Carbery Mattingly, 1809–1839

In 1822, the year of his father's death, while his mother remained gravely ill, young John Mattingly enrolled in a new school, the Washington Catholic Seminary, the forerunner of what is now Gonzaga College. The prestigious school for boys had opened in September 1821 with, according to historian William Warner, a somewhat misleading name because it was "neither exclusively for Catholics nor intended primarily as a seminary for priests."[27] It was immediately successful, enrolling almost 170 students during its first six years. At age fourteen, John was already a proficient scholar of Latin there, winning the premium for the Third Class and *Accesserunt,* or "approaching," in Greek, a second prize shared with another scholar. The *National Intelligencer* of August 1, 1823, gave this notice of his achievement:

> At the late annual examination of the Scholars attending this establishment, the following young gentlemen gave satisfactory proofs of superior diligence and application to their studies.
>
> Classical Department In the Latin Language
> 3d Class
> Mr. John Mattingly, premium
> *Accesserunt:* Robert Barry, Edward Barry
>
> In the Greek language
> 3d class
> Mr. Robert Barry, premium
> *Accesserunt:* Mr. John Mattingly, William Coyle

A year later, on August 2, 1824, six months after Ann Mattingly's dramatic cure, another notice appeared in the *National Intelligencer:* "The Annual Public Examination in this Seminary commenced on the 23d ultimo, and closed on the 28th. In the course of the Examination, the following young gentlemen gave proofs of superior talent and application in the respective Classes to which they belong. Their names are presented to the public as examples for their companions to emulate, and as an encouragement to themselves to continue their laudable exertions in the pursuit of learning." This time, John Mattingly won the premium prize in Greek and *Accesserunt* in Latin. His mother, now healed from her illness, was almost certainly in the audience to watch her son win this prize and to bask in predictions of his future success.

On the last day of his exams, John Mattingly, now age fifteen, was perhaps involved in a famous scuffle that took place between the boys of the Washington Catholic Seminary and Georgetown College and their crosstown rivals, the students of Columbian College, now George Washington University. At Georgetown's annual commencement, on July 28, 1824, the same day young John finished his exams, five hundred people were in the audience in anticipation of a visit by the famous French general Lafayette, who had been invited to tour the United States by President James Monroe. There was to be a reception at the Capitol, and the boys were to take part in the procession. As Georgetown College was the oldest institution of learning in the District of Columbia, it was assigned precedence in the ranks. The Georgetown collegians, joined by students of the Washington Catholic Seminary, took the position assigned to them in the procession. They stood on either side of a central walk that ran through the parade grounds, their place being near the triumphal arch where Lafayette was to enter.

John Gilmary Shea recounts what happened next: "After the distinguished visitor and his *suite* had passed between the ranks of the Georgetown and Washington seminary pupils, they closed together to follow in the procession, when, suddenly, the students of Columbian College, young men of greater age and strength, attempted to prevent them and gain precedence. Georgetown College was not inclined to yield without a struggle, and a collision occurred." The order had been given to advance, and the Columbian boys, bearing a beautiful flag, rushed forward to pass the Georgetown cohort. As they did so, the star on the end of the Columbian banner cut Georgetown's flag from its staff. In an instant, a number of the larger boys, seeing what had been done, made a spring at the Columbian banner and tore it down and bore it off. Shea continues:

> Thus each side lost its colors, but Georgetown maintained its place in the procession, and the students of the college and seminary, led by Rev. Messrs. Levins and Matthews, with the other professors, marched exulting on. Three days after, as a prefect was taking out some of the pupils, they descried their banner hanging from a window of a low frame building on the South side of Bridge Street. They entered the store in the lower part and demanded their property so imperatively that it was restored to them. Upon this, they sent back to Columbian College the trophies which they had carried off. In commemoration of the affair, the Georgetown students had a fine banner painted by an artist named Simpson, representing on one side an eagle with the motto, *Nemini Cedimus,* and the other side the arms of the college.[28]

John Mattingly, being a prize-winning Latin scholar, would have known that the Latin phrase *nemini cedimus* means "yield to no one." In a sense, this motto would become very much his own as he lived out the second half of his short life. It is tempting to speculate what his personal relationship may have been with Rev. Thomas C. Levins, or Democritus. Given the participation of Levins and Matthews in this exciting event with rivals, John likely felt a bond with them. A dynamic, learned teacher like Levins, who read Byron and scoffed at religious enthusiasm, would have been in marked contrast to members of John B. C. Mattingly's very religious family. Given John's ensuing estrangement from his family, Levins's perspective might have been one he embraced.

One of the draft documents about the Mattingly miracle records that his mother's astonishing recovery profoundly affected her fifteen-year-old son. After the healing, according to eyewitnesses, John Mattingly "looked as white as the wall [and declared] no revolution in the nation could have made a deeper impression on his mind."[29] As he finished his final year at the Washington Catholic Seminary, his mother became an object of both public reverence and revulsion. The intense scrutiny of his family, including so much discussion in the press and in the pamphlet war, must have been a source of confusion for John. One might guess that he was under pressure to live up to Carbery expectations.

Six months after the miracle, John entered Georgetown College in September 1824 as a nonpaying student. During this period, students who attended the college tuition-free were typically destined for the priesthood. With relatives already members of religious orders, his aunts who were Carmelites and his uncle Joseph, the Jesuit, it might be expected that Ann Mattingly, the recipient of a stunning grace by virtue of the collaboration of Catholic priests, both in the United States and abroad, would direct her son toward the celibate life of a Roman Catholic priest. A month after John began his studies at the college, Thomas Levins was expelled by his superior from the Jesuits.[30]

Three hundred guests attended Georgetown's commencement of 1825, the end of John's first year at the college, including President John Quincy Adams, Secretary of State Henry Clay, and full representation from the diplomatic core and the army and navy. John Mattingly delivered an oration, "On Medicine," and a poem, "Ode to the Potomac." He also played the "Voice of Hercules" in *Philoctetes—a Tragic Drama*. After the exercises were finished, the *National Journal* reported, "the president of the United States with readiness and satisfaction, at the request of the president of the college, consented to distribute the premiums to those to whom they had been assigned; and if we can augur from the faces of innocent youth, the favor and kind feeling which his benevolent countenance expressed will never be eradicated from their minds." John Mattingly had had an impressive first year at Georgetown and was probably seen as a young man of vast potential at the college. Rev. Stephen Dubuisson became the thirteenth president of Georgetown College in September 1825, but he resigned the following July to go to Rome.[31]

There is no record of John Mattingly returning for a second year at

Georgetown. That autumn, the Georgetown students enjoyed excursions
to Great Falls and to points on the Potomac River. In April 1826, an exhibition was given consisting mainly of declamations and the reading of poems
and other exercises. Several students are mentioned by name as performing, but John is not among them. On July 4, 1826, the college celebrated
Independence Day, holding exercises in the hall. A classmate who had
performed with John in the play the previous year read the Declaration
of Independence. If he was in the audience, John would have heard his
classmate James P. Deery deliver an address on moral purity, three days
before the departure of family friend Rev. Dubuisson for Rome on July 7.[32]

Perhaps Mr. Deery had his former classmate John Mattingly in mind
as he spoke:

> . . . let our vigilance, my fellow students, be unceasing for its
> preservation; let it never be contaminated by the pollution of
> vice; let the cherubim of religion and morality be retained as
> the mercy seat of the Omnipotent; let the steadiness of your vir-
> tue, your perseverant diligence in the acquisition of knowledge,
> be the present harbingers of your future excellence as citizens.
> These are the columns which support the body of freedom's
> fabric. Present habits and associations must form the basis of
> your future character. If eager in the acquisition of knowledge,
> if firm in the practice of duties which religion prescribes, you
> may hereafter be the pride, the support, the ornament of your
> country, the chosen apostles and champion of freedom.[33]

Within a matter of months, John's "habits and associations" and his probable
"pollution of vice" would lead to his sudden departure from Washington.

In a well-known historical coincidence, on that Independence Day in
1826, both John Adams and Thomas Jefferson died; Georgetown students
issued a resolution to wear crape on their left arms for thirty days. Under
these circumstances, the 1826 commencement was a sober event, with
thirty-five students in attendance and eight faculty members, including Rev.

William Feiner, prefect of studies and professor of theology and German, who had just become the college's president; Rev. Francis Dzierozynski, professor of moral philosophy and an enthusiast for the Mattingly miracle; and Brother Joseph Mobberly, who had identified Rev. Levins as the culprit behind the anti-Mattingly miracle tirades in the newspapers two years before. Feiner, a native of Poland, was a man of learning and ability and one of those who came from the Jesuit body in Russia to aid in reorganizing the Society of Jesus in the United States. The college had greatly reduced its cadre of fractious English and American priests. But from the beginning of his presidency, Feiner's health was poor, and he was not able to assume the role with energy and vigor. As Shea wrote about Rev. Feiner, "he failed to obtain much personal influence over the students." With Rev. Dubuisson in Europe, the new Georgetown College president may not have been able to provide John with guidance during a time of crisis in his young life, had John tried to consult him.[34]

The deaths of Adams and Jefferson in 1826 plunged the nation into a period of deep mourning. And although their significant accomplishments were lauded, some may have recalled the infamous poem by Thomas Moore in 1806 that not only slighted the rough-hewn Capital City, but also contained references to Thomas Jefferson's affair with his slave Sally Hemings. Moore had written,

> The weary statesman for repose has fled
> From halls of council to his negro's shed,
> Where blest he woos some black Aspasia's grace
> And dreams of freedom in his slave's embrace![35]

When Ann and John Mattingly removed to Washington from Maryland in 1805 to begin their new life together, they joined thousands, slaves, free blacks, and whites, who were working to raise the Capital City out of the wilderness. This vibrant community of black and white southerners, whose segregation was legislated by complex racial, cultural, and legal divides, in fact commingled in ways that violated some of Washington's most explicit taboos. The Capital City of 1826 was far more cosmopolitan, but the stigma of Jefferson's miscegenation resurfaced when news came of his death. Racial mixing remained an alluring taboo for the young men of Washington.

John did not become a Catholic priest. He did not graduate from Georgetown College and did not live up to the vision of his classmate who encouraged his fellow students to become "the pride, the support, the ornament of your country." During a dramatic period of change within the Carbery household, when Captain Thomas Carbery married Mary H. Manning in 1826, John's relations with the family unraveled. In November of that year, just three months before his eighteenth birthday, John ran away to the frontier town of Moorefield in western Virginia, a remote borderland where even the most forbidden love could find expression.

Moorefield was settled over what Native Americans considered hallowed ground. Their graveyard had been laid out on the floodplain of the river junction, 820 feet above sea level, where the town was located. Two ancient trails—the Seneca and what later became known as the McCullough trader's trail, both following the paths of rivers and crossing the Allegheny divide—also intersected at this plateau. Native Americans had long buried their dead at the crossroads, and the gravesites stretched down to the riverbanks. In the western third of what is now Hardy County, West Virginia, the Moorefield River flows into the south branch of the Potomac. Native Americans cleared large fields for planting in the middle of forests. Well into the twentieth century, these clearings were still called "Indian Old Fields."

Moorefield's limestone soil, rich with Indian bones, arrowheads, and pottery shards, was well suited to growing grass for grazing, corn, and tobacco. As the settlers plowed and built on the floodplain, the ground spit up reminders of the past. A highly finished pipe, with the figure of a snake coiled round the bowl, its head peering over the brim, was found on the riverbank. A human jawbone of enormous size was discovered nearby, with peculiar, prehistoric teeth. It seemed that giants had once roamed this land. This awareness of a long past was woven into the Indian names given to places in the town and perhaps contributed to a culture of tolerance unusual for its day. The 1790 census, for example, lists 411 free, nonwhite people, 42 more than the 369 slaves in the county. At the turn of the nineteenth century, Hardy was apparently the only county in Virginia that had more free black people than slaves. Most of these were likely freed or escaped slaves from Virginia who made their way up the Potomac River Valley to the mountainous border country. People of African origins living in Hardy County could see that more than half of their number had escaped the chains of slavery. To the nineteenth-century mind, Moorefield was a town wrested from savages and reclaimed from the wilderness. The dangers and attractions of the frontier lay to the west. This borderland enticed nonconformists seeking freedom and individual expression in the vast wilderness spaces.[36]

In 1826, young John B. C. Mattingly abandoned his studies at Georgetown College, jettisoned his training for the priesthood, and eloped to the borderland with Harriet Doyle, who was pregnant with their first son. Thomas Joseph Mattingly was born on June 2, 1827, in Moorefield. Whether the couple was married in a civil ceremony or by a Catholic priest is not recorded, and John's mother was not a guest at the nuptials. Her shock and disappointment at John's recklessness was acute, and her worst fears had been realized. John had done more than throw away a promising future; he had abandoned moral principles. What John had done was, in his family's view, unforgivable. He had contaminated the family line by marrying a woman who was far below the social standing of the Carberys. Furthermore, Harriet Doyle was, in the nineteenth-century definition, almost certainly "colored," and therefore, so was Ann Mattingly's first grandson.

John had left his family in Washington suddenly and without explanation, and they may not have been aware of this relationship. Harriet has remained fairly elusive, but her father, Martin Doyle, had been involved in an insolvent debtor's case in Maryland in 1802. The 1827 Washington directory lists his address simply as "canal wharf, eastern branch." He seems to have been a dockworker on the Washington City Canal, which connected the Anacostia River to Tiber Creek and the Potomac. This canal was a mile-and-a-half trench cut out of Tiber Creek that flowed along what is now the National Mall along Constitution Avenue. Thomas Carbery, as we have seen, was one of the investors and had a wharf nearby.

According to historian John Wennersten, the Washington City Canal after 1810 was the major construction project in the District of Columbia in which Irish workers were involved. Those workers, many of whom were imported for the job, endured poor food, miserable wages, and unsanitary living conditions. Riots over wages sometimes broke out among them, and canal workers were widely feared in the city. Public drunkenness of the canal workers also contributed to their violence. When the canal opened in 1815, only barges drawing three feet could navigate it. The wooden lining and pilings were poorly maintained and rotted. Wennersten also writes that there was a large population of blacks, bondsmen and free, living in the canal area at this time. Martin Doyle was known to have been in Baltimore County, Maryland, during 1802, and a number of Maryland citizens moved to the Federal City to work. Of Harriet's mother, little is known. It appears that John Baptist Carbery Mattingly fell in love with a young woman well below his station and expectations, and that they fled to western Virginia to cover up a pregnancy and illegitimate birth.[37]

In a letter dated Washington City, May 16, 1828, Captain Thomas Carbery wrote to Rev. Dubuisson in Rome: "We had not heard from John Mattingly for 18 months, till a few days ago and then only saw a letter to William Barryman. He is at Weston, in the back part of Virginia, where, he says, that he writes in the clerk's office and is doing very well. He seems to be penitent and promises to write to his mother. As both her and myself have written to him, we may expect to hear from him, direct, in a few days. The manner in which he went off has given his mother and indeed the whole family great uneasiness, but I hope his future good conduct will make amends for it."[38] No evidence has surfaced of John's work in Weston, but the baby was born in Moorefield, more than one hundred miles away, according to the obituary of Thomas Joseph Mattingly.

Thomas Carbery's mention of John's disappearance comes in a long, newsy letter that details the establishment of a holiday on the anniversary of Mrs. Mattingly's cure on March 10, 1824. This anniversary was celebrated annually at St. Patrick's Church with a 7:00 A.M. Mass. "We celebrated the Tenth of March as when you were with us and shall continue to do so as long as we live," Carbery wrote to Dubuisson. "It is a day of great glory in the Annals of Catholick America; to us particularly and to me especially. Those feelings and appearances, which you do justly describe, made too strong an impression upon me to be forgotten . . . I cannot conceive of any exhibition of God's power upon earth could make a greater impression upon me than did the instantaneous restoration of my Sister from her bed of sickness and who, but a moment before, was a map of the most filthy sickening corruption. 'Nothing is hard or impossible to God.'" Thomas Carbery here underscores his determination to keep the miracle, and his sister, prominently in the public eye.

The language is striking in its immediacy; four years after the event, the cure was still very much a central part of their lives. Carbery continued, drawing a comparison between the situation of Ann Mattingly and Lazarus being raised from the tomb: "How different was the situation of Mrs. Mattingly. She was not dead, it is true, but she was infinitely beyond restoration, from human skills. In her, all that complicate machinery of the system was rent asunder, her lungs devoured and her body a heap of putrification. She, who could not, for all the Kingdoms of the Earth, a moment before her cure, raise her hand from the bed, or speak above a whisper, so weak or seldom to be heard, even with the ear to her mouth." Carbery concludes that Mrs. Mattingly's cure was even more miraculous than Lazarus's. Mrs. Mattingly was still enjoying robust health, and the family was celebrating the miracle with solemn devotion—but this time, without John.

Well into this letter, after a lengthy discussion of the miracle and the possible reassignment of Rev. Matthews from the parish, Carbery mentions that he himself had been married on November 20, 1826, to Miss Mary H. Manning of Virginia. The November date approximates the date of John's departure. Was this wedding the catalyst of John's leaving? Carbery's letter mentions the eighteen-month time frame, so it is possible that the family gathering was an impetus. Carbery added: "Our son Henry, about eight months old, I have dedicated to that honorable and distinguished S.J. [So-

ciety of Jesus] of which you are a member and to which I am so much attached. May he live to join it and comply with all its precepts. . . . With the
exception of my marriage, we are exactly as you left us, even to old Hanna.
We all live together, at the same place, and in the most perfect harmony of
good feeling." Right after this section of the letter, in which he dedicates his
eight-month-old son to the Jesuits, Thomas Carbery reveals the breach with
John Mattingly—a singular example of a lack of "perfect harmony" in the
household. John, with his free tuition at Georgetown, had not done as his
family wished and entered the priesthood. Instead, he had run away to the
wilderness of western Virginia. Carbery then reports on two of the former
Jesuits who had taken adversarial positions on the Mattingly miracle, Rev.
Baxter and Rev. Levins, both of whom subsequently left the society. Baxter
had died in Philadelphia, and Levins was moved to New York.

A few days after her brother Thomas wrote this letter, Ann Mattingly
also wrote to Rev. Dubuisson: "Oh my Father, pray for me, and for my dear
children. Brother has written to you concerning my dear John & I hope
all from the mercy & merits of my Jesus. Susan continues to enjoy good
health & with gratitude I can say she is a good child." Ann Mattingly's letter
merely alludes to John's disappearance, contrasting him with her "good"
child Susan; the bulk of it is a passionate expression of her love for God
and her fervent wish to enter a convent. She writes, "I have no wish but
that God's will may be accomplished yet the desire of leaving the world
presses me, yet I know it is in obedience alone I can know the will of my
God and as long as my Confessor sees proper to keep me where I am &
rest satisfied." She adds, "every day this earth becomes more contemptible
& my desire of an Eternal union with my Jesus more ardent yet in all his
will, his will, his adorable will [is] my only wish, as it is this alone, that can
make me happy here & hereafter." Even with a second chance at life, Ann
Mattingly was not allowed by her priests, Stephen Dubuisson and William
Matthews, to make her own choices. Her letter to Dubuisson suggests that
she understands and struggles to accept her role to live as a laywoman in
the world. In a curious statement, she speaks about her own body in the
third person, as if it were somehow distanced from her true self: "Now as

to the poor body, it remains as strong as the first moment that it was cured [and] the allpowerful hand that touched it still supports it & the attention & respect I continue to receive only serves to humble & make me dread the least offense."[39]

In this letter, Mrs. Mattingly writes most fervently, not about her heartbreak over the rift with her son, but about her powerful attraction to the Holy Eucharist. She describes her intense fear and dread of the majesty of God as she approaches the sacrament, depicting herself shrinking up "to nothing" in awe. Her spirituality is expressed in the following passionate terms: "Yet I feel a longing desire to be united to him, & who can express his infinite goodness mercy & love when on receiving him he is pleased as it was to overpower me with a sweetness inexpressible, it appears & really leaves in my mouth a licquor of sweetness which I swallow as if poured in my mouth by large draughts. My hands face & vail is [*sic*] sometimes perfumed with the smell which to my heart and soul is inexpressible. What is [it] I say? My God is it you[?], my fear of being deluded is great & my own unworthiness is ever present to me." Dubuisson copied this letter and sent it to Bishop England as evidence for the second set of affidavits concerning the miracle published in 1830. Today, we recognize it as the eroticized language used by mystics to describe an ecstatic experience of God.[40]

What is striking about Ann Mattingly's letter, as well as Thomas Carbery's, is the intense focus on the spiritual and lack of concentration on the domestic. In the letter to their priest and close family friend, John's disappearance merits scant attention. It is doubtful that at this point, the family knew the full extent of his transgression or that a child had been born to him and Harriet Doyle. Both letters speak of hope for reconciliation with John, suggesting that they had not yet discovered what would become for them an irreconcilable breach.

In crossing the Appalachian Mountains into western Virginia, John Mattingly for a time disappeared into the frontier, a place that historian John R. Dichtl has characterized as "both frightening and thrilling, a contested space of challenges and possibilities." Dichtl examines the frontier as a place where Catholics mixed with non-Catholics in a hinterland removed from the control and surveillance of Catholic authorities. He notes that in 1821, for example, Charles Nerinckx, a frontier priest in Kentucky, wrote to Cardinal Francesco Luigi Fontana in Rome asking for guidance on the treatment of "couples who had eloped and were married by non-Catholic ministers. What sins did they commit and censures did they incur? Should the couple or those 'who welcome the returning couple into their home' be denied entrance into the church on Sundays? Should they be allowed 'to assist at sacred functions' if they wanted to be reconciled with the church and while they are waiting to be reconciled?"[41] Nerinckx's questions demonstrate that John's elopement, in the view of the Roman Catholic Church, put in peril not only his own soul, but also those of his family should they become reconciled to his actions. Furthermore, John's defiance of the powerful Carbery family culture suggests that Georgetown College's motto of unwillingness to yield to anyone in a contest—*nemini cedimus*—is an apt descriptor of his character.

In the 1830 Georgetown census, a family of "Jno Mattingly" appears that closely matches what we know about John Baptist Carbery Mattingly: the family includes one male aged twenty to thirty (John would be twenty-one in 1830); one female, also aged twenty to thirty; one male child younger than five (Thomas Joseph would be three years old in 1830), and one female child younger than five (John and Harriet's second child, Annie Elizabeth, was born about 1830). Thomas Joseph Mattingly recalled that he moved back to Washington at about age three, so the timeline matches other information we have about the family. In the same census the family of Thomas Carbery no longer includes Ann, who would have been forty-six years old and who, during this period, spent long periods of time at the Georgetown Visitation Monastery.[42]

John Baptist Carbery Mattingly returned to Washington about 1830, just as Bishop England's second pamphlet on his mother's miraculous cure in 1824 was appearing. But in a letter that Ann Mattingly wrote to Stephen Dubuisson dated August 5, 1830, she makes no mention of John, writing generally, "All our family likewise desires to be most kindly & respectfully remembered to you and beg your blessing also."[43] John's sister, Mary Susan, likely pleased her mother and the Carberys by making an advantageous marriage to a Washington lawyer, Richard Lay, on January 9, 1832. Thus a clear divide was established between the two children of Ann and John Mattingly.

In the months before Susan's wedding, John was struggling greatly to support his wife Harriet and little Thomas Joseph and Annie Elizabeth, who were likely named after their great-uncles and grandmother. Like his father before him, it appears that John was falling into deep debt. A small notice appeared in the *National Intelligencer* in September 1831: "For sale at public auction: brown mare, at the Centre Mket Hose, [for keeping,] I placed in my stable, as the prop of John Mattingly, —Wm Samuels." At some point that year, John Baptist Carbery Mattingly, like his father, was imprisoned for debt. He appeared in court on February 29, 1832 (a leap year), and affirmed that he was for some uncertain time committed to the Washington jail after his father-in-law, Martin Doyle, had filed a suit against him. In court papers his real property holdings are listed as "none," and the amount due his father-in-law is $19.92, a little more than $500 in today's currency. In addition to Doyle, a list of thirty-eight other creditors is attached. Significantly, among them are half a dozen doctors. Given the Mattingly family's genetic predisposition to early-onset ALS4, the large number of doctors among John's creditors suggests he may have been suffering from the creeping paralysis.[44]

Many other creditors were tavern owners, which help paint a picture of a family sinking into despair. While the Carbery family celebrated Susan's marriage in January 1832, John was probably in debtor's prison. Merritt Tarleton, a tavern owner, paid John's bail of $100 (about $2,500 today). Also one of John's creditors, he must have taken pity on either John or his impoverished wife and children and was appointed trustee of all John's worldly possessions for the amount of one dollar. Significantly, neither the Carbery family nor Martin Doyle paid John's bail. Thomas and James Carbery also appear on the long list of creditors, but the family rupture seems to have been complete by this time. On Thursday, March 1, 1832, a notice was published in the *National Intelligencer* that John Mattingly, among other insolvent debtors, had applied to be discharged from prison.[45]

John Baptist Carbery Mattingly was released from debtor's prison eight years after the first miraculous cure of his mother, and one year after the second. Nine months later, Harriet Doyle Mattingly gave birth to a son, John, born on December 6, 1832. This child survived until at least August 23, 1833, when he was baptized at St. Patrick's Church in Washington. The fact that it was a Catholic baptism is significant, because clearly, John and Harriet had not left the church. The family breach, then, had origins other than merely a difference of religion. Presumably, John and Harriet's baby did not survive into adulthood, because no subsequent record of him has been found. This baptismal record is also the last known historical trace of Ann's son, John Baptist Carbery Mattingly. We do not know whether he succumbed to the deterioration of ALS4 or perhaps of alcoholism, given his record of debt in taverns. In the city of Washington during 1839, John was one of 372 people who died—twenty-one of them from drunkenness. The final story of John's death remains a mystery that so far is accurately characterized by the maxim "Yield to no one."[46]

More Hohenlohe Miracles, 1824–1838

During the period that John was sinking deeper into desperation, Bishop John England publicly tackled a question that was under discussion by nineteenth-century theologians: whether or not miracles can occur in an age other than that lived by Jesus Christ. "We ought to examine every alleged miracle," England wrote, "whether of the first or of the nineteenth century . . . we have no power to tell the Almighty that he shall not make a revelation to us at one time, as well as another; and I assert that the proof of the truth of the miracle is to be found in its own nature, and not in the circumstances of the time at which it was wrought. There is nothing in the nature of things, or in the nature of religion to make it impossible for God to do now works similar to those done by him at any former time."[47] England clearly thought that the age of miracles continued into his own time, and several other seemingly supernatural events occurred that appeared to give credence to his views.

The attention given to the Mattingly miracle of 1824 created immense interest in the favors of Prince Hohenlohe during 1824–1831, and numerous additional cures occurred in the archdiocese of Baltimore. These included M. L. Chevigne, a mathematics professor at St. Mary's College, who was restored to health in 1824; Sister Beatrix Meyers of the Georgetown Visitation Monastery, healed on February 10, 1825; Sister Benedicta Parsons of the Sisters of Charity of Emmitsburg, healed on June 20, 1826; Sister Josephine Collins, also of Emmitsburg, healed on August 20, 1826; and Sister Mary Apollonia Digges of the Visitation Monastery, healed on January 21, 1831.

Chevigne, one of the few male miraculés, was a native of Nantes who during the French Revolution entered the British Navy as a captain. In 1795, he moved to the United States and began teaching mathematics at St. Mary's College. When he decided to follow Prince's Hohenlohe's regimen in 1824, he had been in poor health for nearly twenty-five years, having developed in 1799 a mysterious illness that created a tremendous appetite. He was compelled to eat as many as ten meals a day. In 1812, he suffered an attack of fever and discharge of blood from the mouth. His physicians prescribed a bland diet of mush made out of rye flour, molasses, and milk. This diet moderated the symptoms, which he described: "When the want of eating became violent, I felt a twitching accompanied by a cough, which ceased as soon as I took some food, and the throwing up of blood . . . proceeded from the acrid humour; this frequently occurred but in small quantities. Another effect of this disease when I delayed taking food, was to contract my stomach so much as to cause a difficulty of breathing, so that I used to say that it was impossible for me to fast, as to exist without breathing."[48] It is interesting that the only documented cure of a man by Prince Hohenlohe in North America appears to be of some sort of eating disorder, which today is more typically associated with women.

The first novena on Chevigne's behalf was made in February 1824, then again in March and April. On April 10, Chevigne arose at 2:00 A.M. to attend a Mass timed, as they erroneously believed, with the prince's morning Mass in Bamberg. He then went back to bed until it was time for

morning Mass at the college. He fasted until lunchtime, when he ate a dinner of fish and vegetables. He then found his symptoms were gone. He was
reticent to share the details of his cure, but eventually they were published
in Bishop England's *Catholic Miscellany*, accompanied by an affidavit from
his physician, Dr. Peter Chotard, who had written to Stephen Dubuisson
that Mrs. Mattingly's cure was evidence of the "finger of God." Chevigne's
cure was short-lived, however; he died two years later in 1826.

Sister Beatrix Meyers also experienced a miraculous cure that was
credited to Prince Hohenlohe. The twenty-seven-year-old nun had become
ill with violent headaches and a general weakness. By September 1825, it
appeared she was dying. Extreme Unction, the anointing of the dying, had
been administered, and she remained ill until January. Her confessor, the
French Jesuit Rev. Joseph-Pierre Picot Clorivière, was confident that she
would be cured through the intersession of Prince Hohenlohe. On February
1, 1825, a novena was begun for Sister Beatrix and three other sick Visi-
tandine sisters. On February 10 at three o'clock in the morning, Clorivière
brought Communion to the four sisters in the infirmary. Suddenly, Sister
Beatrix called out to her superior: "Mother! Mother, I think I am cured.
Lord Jesus, may thy name be glorified forever!" Her Protestant physician,
Dr. Benjamin Bohrer, was startled to see her sitting in the convent parlor,
completely well. She continued in good health for another ten years and
died in 1843.[49]

Priests and superiors purposely downplayed Prince Hohenlohe's
purported cure of Sister Benedicta Parsons at Emmitsburg on June 20,
1826. With the permission of their confessor, Mother Rose White wrote to
the archbishop detailing Sister Benedicta's severe illness and astonishing
recovery: "Our Reverend Superior thinks that whilst we ought not hesi-
tate with your approbation to publish to our friends the infinite mercies of
God—yet ought to avoid any publication in print, which is unnecessary
now after Mrs. Mattingly's case has been fully published—it might appear
in us seeking self glory, also such publications would require affidavits etc.
etc. which would draw our Sisters from the obscurity in which they ought
to remain as much as possible." Mother Rose carefully assessed the pros

and cons of the publicity surrounding Mrs. Mattingly's cure and opted to preserve the privacy of her community. Two months later, a second cure attributed to Prince Hohenlohe occurred at Emmitsburg, of Sister Josephine Collins. Mother Rose again wrote to Archbishop Maréchal to inform him of the cure. A year later, Sister Josephine herself wrote to the archbishop, asking that her identity be kept confidential.[50]

Another well-documented cure credited to Prince Hohenlohe occurred ten days before Ann Mattingly's second dramatic healing in 1831. Sister Mary Apollonia Digges, of the Georgetown Visitation Monastery, had been diagnosed with pulmonary consumption, or tuberculosis. On January 10 the convent community began a novena in union with Prince Hohenlohe. Rev. Dubuisson had returned from Rome and again followed the directions for the novena and Mass. A few minutes after receiving communion, Sister Apollonia exclaimed: "Jesus! Jesus! My God! Thou art all mine, and I am entirely thine!" She reported that following the reception of the Eucharist, she had been pervaded with a feeling of well-being. Once again, Dubuisson found himself a witness to a miraculous cure. The sister had seemingly boundless energy after the cure, picking up chairs to prove her strength, running to visit the sisters in other parts of the convent, and eating baked apples and pound cake. Mrs. Mattingly gave an affidavit of the cure of Sister Apollonia in February 1831 before Justice of the Peace Charles W. H. Wharton. Sister Apollonia, understanding that the gender of those cured was perceived as undermining the power of the miracles, commented that it would be important to pray for cures of men. She died at age eighty-nine, fifty-eight years after her sudden cure by Prince Hohenlohe.[51]

In the Georgetown Visitation Monastery, six miraculous cures occurred between 1825 and 1838, three of which were attributed to Prince Hohenlohe and three to the application of a miraculous medal. Three cures occurred at St. Joseph's Convent in Emmitsburg, Maryland; two among the Sisters of Charity of Nazareth in Kentucky; and one in the Carmelite monastery at Portobacco, Maryland. Curran has observed that with the exception of the Carmelite community, all these religious orders had connections with French Jesuits or Sulpicians. At the time of their cures, the nuns ranged in age from 20 to 49 years, with the median age 37 and the average 34.5. Curran notes that the gender domination of females in the miraculous cures was not peculiar to the United States. The high percentage of nuns among the cured was, however, an American Catholic phenomenon. Rev. Clorivière, in the tradition of Stephen Dubuisson, was also a promoter of the power of these North American miracles, stating, "The object of God in working these miracles—so multiple—so public—so incontestable—is to preserve his Church—in showing his predilection & preference for her—over all other churches which are not his & can never please him."[52]

For his part, Dubuisson continued to champion the power of Prince Hohenlohe's miracles until the 1860s, underscoring the priest's role as a conduit for God's grace. About Sister Apollonia, who lifted twenty-eight-pound weights to demonstrate her gift of extraordinary strength after her miraculous healing, Dubuisson wrote, "When it is observed that the person has not only been brought back to the integrity of health, but is now found to possess physical, bodily forces which she never had before,—forces far surpassing what is ordinarily possessed by individuals of the same sex and complexion,—forces that endure, that bear any test,—then, indeed, the mind, overwhelmed, cannot resist the inference, *Digitus Dei est hic*." With this affirmation that "the finger of God is here," Dubuisson articulated his vision that the male priesthood functions well as an intermediary by which God can improve on the female body.[53]

Mrs. Mattingly's Foot

On July 15, 1830, Bishop John England's *Examination of Evidence Reported to the Archbishop of Baltimore, upon the Restoration of Mrs. Ann Mattingly* was published in Washington to be sold for a price of fifty cents. Six years after the miraculous cure, there was still active interest in the Federal City, and Captain Thomas Carbery had planned yearly commemorations of it. Just after Thanksgiving 1830, on November 29, Ann Mattingly had paid a visit to the home of the Sisters of Charity in Washington. On her way to Mass at St. Patrick's, she fell down and her leg and foot were twisted under her body. She could not return home that day because of the intense swelling. The next day, Mrs. Mattingly tried to walk back to her brother's house half a mile away. It took her two hours to hobble home in excruciating pain. This exertion caused the ankle to balloon, and her whole foot turned a deep purple. As Christmas approached, she was still unable to walk. She returned to Georgetown Visitation Monastery in a carriage for the holiday, intending to attend Mass in the convent chapel.

Mrs. Mattingly was carried to a cell near the novitiate that had been assigned to her. The convent's physician, the Protestant Dr. Bohrer, who had treated several of the nuns who were later miraculously cured, was unable to help Mrs. Mattingly's foot. In fact, the swelling now reached to her hip, and the doctor recommended application of a large number of leeches. According to an affidavit, Mrs. Mattingly's foot was "swollen to deformity, with the sinews and veins apparently distended, and the color extremely dark, to half way up the leg." This was a probable case of gangrene, which Dr. Bohrer pronounced could "not be trifled with." Mrs. Mattingly applied some of the palliative remedies that had afforded her some relief. Then she observed to the sisters that she would put her confidence in God and "make use of all the faith she possessed." She believed that "mortification," or a dangerous infection, was setting in. In 1831, such an untreated infection could result in death.[54]

Mrs. Mattingly, however, did not pray in union with her former savior, Prince Hohenlohe. Instead, she put her confidence directly in the Blessed Virgin Mary, that through her intercession, she might obtain from God either relief or the necessary grace to die a happy death. Within thirty minutes, she felt relief: "A sensation of softness succeeded to the former most painful rigidity; she drew up her foot; pressed it with her hand,—then raised, with that same foot, the whole of the bed covering (six blankets and a thick counterpane)—and, to use the familiar term, *tucked it around,* without any pain or difficulty."[55] All pain had left her, and her foot and limb had recovered their natural strength.

The next morning, she joined the sisters in the chapel for Mass, much to their surprise. Mrs. Mattingly had experienced a second miraculous cure, and a new set of affidavits was produced. Once again, she found herself to be the talk of Washington. About two dozen Visitation sisters swore affidavits, as well as Stephen Dubuisson, Captain Thomas Carbery and his wife, and Mrs. Mattingly's sisters, Ruth and Catharine. Rev. Matthews and Dr. Bohrer also appeared in court to provide witness. Susan, soon to be married, did not appear, and, of course, neither did John. Ann Mattingly's turn to the Blessed Virgin Mary for help was a harbinger of a rise in Catholic devotion to Mary during the mid-nineteenth century. After this miracle, something of a breach occurred between Ann Mattingly and Stephen Dubuisson, who actively promoted the role of the priesthood in miracles throughout the 1830s. Whether this breach resulted from Mrs. Mattingly's dispensing of the priest as an intermediary in miracles or from her persistence in wanting to join the Visitation community, or both, is not clear.

On April 16, 1831, Ann Mattingly wrote to Rev. Dubuisson from the Visitation Monastery, and she was clearly upset: "I speak plainly, as you know, I repose entire confidence in you—then, I think your letter [of March 22, 1831] was too cold. I know that I do not merit the affection of any one, still, to be treated coolly by one whom I consider as a *true Father,* is more than my humility can bear. However, this neither does nor shall diminish my filial affection for you, I shall ever consider myself *your child* even if you do not deign to call me so. I am afraid you have no mind to acknowledge me such. You may be assured that a little word of advice from you, would have soothed me in my present state, but I suppose dereliction is my position, and I must submit."[56] The discussion of dereliction suggests she had swerved from some duty in the eyes of her confessor.

After noting that one of the Georgetown Visitation sisters, Sister Gertrude, had left the convent, Mrs. Mattingly continued: "Oh that it were in my power to embrace what she has renounced! But, I am not without hope although it is about the eleventh hour for me. I may still be called." She concludes the letter with this plaintive appeal: "Do, my dear Father, write a little more affectionately, & call me your child, or your unworthy child, just as you please. At any rate, write." She then confesses her anger that

Dubuisson called her "Madam," saying "I *am mad* at it." In a note appended to the letter, Sister Mary Augustine wrote in French that "despite the sorrow that has tested her, her greatest concern has been to place her entire confidence in your charity." Mrs. Mattingly does not seem to be alluding to family troubles here, although they may be in the background of Sister Mary Augustine's comment. Perhaps Dubuisson did not fully approve of the handling of the cure of her foot and inquired specifically about the pamphlet to be published. As did many of the continental Jesuit priests, Dubuisson wished to keep the power of the priesthood as a central feature of miraculous cures, and Mrs. Mattingly's self-cure in many ways undermined his efforts. The privileging of a Hohenlohe cure over a self-cure may be seen in a letter sent from Archbishop James Whitfield, Maréchal's successor, to Stephen Dubuisson in July 1831. The letter discusses at length the cure of Sister Mary Apollonia and encourages Dubuisson to document the miracle. The cure of Mrs. Mattingly's foot merits only a single sentence.[57]

An undated document with a cover page in the hand of Dubuisson—entitled "Prayers recited by Mrs. Ann Mattingly before and after the cure of her foot, which took place on the 1st of January 1831, at about 10 1/2 at night, in the Convent of Visitation . . . of Georgetown, D.C."—presents us with a window into the mind of Ann Mattingly at age forty-seven. If Dubuisson asked her to write down the prayer that she said before and after her cure, as we might surmise, Mrs. Mattingly complied with an outpouring. The cover sheet is appended with a ribbon to seventeen pages in her distinctive script, a direct appeal to the Blessed Virgin to intercede with God on her behalf. Mrs. Mattingly's neat, straight penmanship is in the ornate practiced and slanted style of the day. Though most of the language of the prayer is conventional, some of it is extremely passionate and personal.

In the prayer called "Thanksgiving" she writes: "Oh, my God! Oh my Lord! Oh my Maker! Oh my Redeemer! Oh my Benefactor! Oh my best friend! My most loving Father! My joy, my comfort, my hope, my love, my all! I adore thee, I honour & love thee with my whole heart, with my whole soul, & with all my senses, with all of my strength, with all my powers, faculties and senses, with all my capacity and ability, and I ardently desire

to increase in thy love every moment of my life and during all eternity."
Mrs. Mattingly was now living in the wake of her second cure, having seem-
ingly cheated death twice. She clearly expressed a desire to become a bride
of Christ and live out her life within the peaceful walls of the Visitation
Monastery. But not wanting to be derelict in any of her duties, and mind-
ful of her brother's and her priests' wishes, she remained in the world.
In 1833, Thomas Carbery gave another of his commemorative dinners on
March 10, and a transcript of a toast to Mrs. Mattingly in French remains:
"Heureuse Mattingly, ton sont digne d'envie / Puisse-t-il exciter un élan
généreuse [Happy Mattingly, worthy of envy for this surge of generosity]!"
The toastmaster urges "Heureuse Mattingly" to "teach all mortals to live for
Heaven" and to further "elevate herself, to fly toward the throne of heaven."
The toastmaster captured what she must have felt was truly an enormous
burden for a woman about to turn fifty.[58]

Despite the fame that engulfed her after both the 1824 and 1831 miraculous cures, Ann Mattingly was an intensely private woman, a person
who yearned to escape the spotlight. Her own family tragedies—her separation from her husband and estrangement from her son—became subli-
mated to the mythic role she felt compelled to assume. Having weathered
devastating personal losses and seeking spiritual comfort, Mrs. Mattingly
longed to enter religious life and flee the world. But her brother, Thomas;
Rev. Dubuisson; and her confessor, Father Matthews, worked to persuade
her that she should not, as they put it, hide her light under a bushel. It was
God's will, they told her, to be the prominent laywoman whom Prince Hohenlohe had cured. By living in the world, not in a convent, Ann Mattingly
was an embodiment of the word of God for the growing American Catholic
Church. Rose Hawthorne Lathrop, daughter of Nathaniel Hawthorne and
now herself a candidate for Catholic sainthood, wrote of Mrs. Mattingly's
sacrifice: "It seems to us that Mrs. Mattingly . . . who could not seclude
herself in the cloistered life, though she desired to—was destined to become and to remain an example and a living instance, to every one, of the
doctrine and mystery of the Holy Eucharist, at the moment when she was
restored to health, after receiving the real yet glorified body of our Lord,

in the consecrated wafer." Lathrop captures the forging of Mrs. Mattingly's iconic role that has until now obscured the details of her personal life. In a letter to a fellow priest in July 1835, Rev. Stephen Dubuisson concisely summed up what the role of "Miracle Ann" was to be for the remainder of her life: "Mrs. Mattingly likewise continues the living miracle."[59]

SEVEN

Conclusion

Thus quickly do miracles sometimes come to pass; the moment they have
occurred, they at once take their place, with all their supernatural quality,
in the natural course of things. And the stream which we choose to call Time—
we, who so easily obscure the fact that it belongs to the current of Eternity—
goes flowing on, with or past the miracles. And sometimes they are
remembered, and sometimes forgotten.

—Rose Hawthorne Lathrop, *A Story of Courage* (1895)

The Carberys, the Mattinglys, and Me: Visitation Monastery, Georgetown, April 2006

The monastery archivist had just finished her presentation to alumnae of
the venerable Georgetown Visitation Preparatory School, updating them
on recent initiatives at the Catholic girls' high school and on the planned
renovations of the campus, including the archives. The talk was part of a
fund-raising effort for alums, and the archivist happened to mention that
a professor had been doing some research in the Visitation archives for a
book on the Mattingly miracle. The previous summer, the archivist and
other religious women at Visitation had hosted me, the professor, for four
nights in the Hermitage, a little apartment that had once been part of the
school's dormitory. I had studied letters, annals, and other convent records
about miracles at the monastery and conducted research at other archives in
Washington, D.C. I was thrilled to be a guest where Ann Mattingly herself
had found some measure of peace.

Each night, after a day of research in the city, I would return to the
convent and pass through the ornate iron gates that set the grounds apart
from the rest of the world. I would wave to the guard in the little sentry
house, take the elevator to the second floor, and walk down a long passage-

way connecting an empty classroom building to the former dormitory in a very old section of the compound. The monastery was in a separate area of the property, so once I entered the apartment, I was alone in this inner sanctum. In the silence of the convent, I felt intensely connected to the history of this place that dated back to the turn of the nineteenth century and whose motto is "Educating women of faith, vision, and purpose since 1799." My isolation in a secluded part of the monastery was an unfamiliar feeling, since my own home is a bustling household with a husband, two sons, and a high-spirited dog. The deep quiet of being cloistered and far away from everyone else inside the compound by the length of two empty buildings gave me an amazing sense of safety and peace.

For more than 210 years, Visitation sisters and their students have inhabited this sacred ground. When Washington, D.C., was burned in August 1814, the sisters nursed soldiers wounded in defense of the capital. During the two centuries of its existence, hundreds of people, undoubtedly some soldiers, some students, and many sisters, had breathed their last here. In the graveyard outside, generations of women religious rested in peace after passing their lives almost entirely within these cloistered walls. Ann Mattingly had spent several seasons here, and she felt a lifelong affection for this place. In the old dormitory where I was staying, generations of adolescent hilarity had pealed, and heartbreak had been sobbed into a pillow. When I turned out the lights and climbed into the narrow single bed, all was utter silence. C. S. Lewis's friend, the woman who did not believe in ghosts, would not have expected to see one here, but other people might. I did not see a ghost in the old dormitory, but that doesn't mean that extraordinary things didn't happen in the monastery.

When the archivist finished her talk to the audience of alumnae, a remarkable coincidence occurred. As Bishop John England observed, "We have no power to tell the Almighty that he shall not make a revelation to us at one time, as well as another." Coincidences are not miracles, and generations of Carberys and Mattinglys had continuing relationships with the Visitation Monastery, but what happened next was revelatory, at least to me. The archivist told me that after her talk, an elderly woman approached her,

and introduced herself as a direct Carbery descendent. The woman said
that "something was troubling her, that she had a box of letters and assorted
papers, some of them Ann Mattingly's, and she wondered if I would want
to see them. I said I did, and asked permission to tell you about them
also."[1]

Following this tip, I contacted Mrs. Williams, launching a friendship with Ann Mattingly's then eighty-four-year-old great-great-great-niece,
whose important collection of family materials has been an invaluable resource for this book. Mrs. Williams and I talked on the phone, and she
invited me not only to see the collection, but to stay with her if I so wished.
I went to Washington, D.C., in June 2006 with my scanner and slept on
couch cushions on the floor of the apartment of a total stranger. We became collaborators in unraveling the mysteries of the Mattingly family.
Mrs. Williams's collection includes letters, photos, scrapbooks, and other
materials. For this book, perhaps, the most significant material in the collection were transcriptions from the now-lost Carbery Bible that had been
given to Bishop Philip M. Hannan in 1965 by Mrs. Mattingly's great-great-
granddaughter, Mrs. Robert L. Walsh. An uncle of Mrs. Williams had been
interested in genealogy and had transcribed birth and death dates from the
Bible. This was fortunate, because authorities at St. Patrick's Church now
have no record of the Bible, which they say has been lost.[2]

I had already been in contact, since about 2003, with one of Ann
Mattingly's great-great-great-granddaughters, Mrs. Clarke, herself an accomplished genealogist. Mrs. Clarke is descended directly from John and
Harriet Mattingly. We have worked closely together to solve the many family
mysteries. I have also met two great-great-great-nephews of Ann Mattingly,
and each of these descendents has provided me with invaluable material and
insight into her story. Miracles are not the same as coincidences. But who
is to say that the encounters we pass off as happenstance are not revelations
of the interconnectedness that binds us all in the web of history?

"Yield to No One": John Baptist Carbery Mattingly's Secret

Mrs. Clarke is a trim, fair-skinned grandmother with dancing blue eyes, hearkening back to an Irish heritage. Her passions include her large family and genealogy. For years, she had puzzled over the elusiveness of Ann's husband, John Mattingly, and their son, John Baptist Carbery Mattingly. Why were they so hard to track through genealogy's usual paths? And why did her great-great-great-grandmother, Ann Mattingly, and her wealthy great-great-great-uncle, Captain Thomas Carbery, make a complete break with John Baptist Carbery Mattingly and his family? Ann and John Mattingly's son, according to material in Mrs. Williams's family collection, died in August 1839 at age thirty. No other record of his death or burial has been found.

A woman named Harriet Mattingly died ten years later in the Mt. Airy district of Washington, D.C. She had lived at the corner of Sixth and H Streets, not far from the original Carbery house on Sixth Street that had been built after the family had moved to the Capital City from St. Mary's County about 1805. According to newspaper accounts and records of the Congressional Cemetery, Harriet Mattingly's body was taken from the home of her son and buried in the Congressional Cemetery in 1849. The two surviving children of John B. C. Mattingly and Harriet, Ann's grandchildren, were Thomas Joseph and Annie Elizabeth Mattingly, both of whom were born in Moorefield, West Virginia. When their father died in 1839, Thomas was twelve years old and Annie Elizabeth was about nine. The family had returned to the Federal City from West Virginia about 1830, and they appear in the 1830 census. Ten years later, the 1840 census lists a "Harriot" Mattingly, age thirty to forty, living in Washington City with a son, age ten to fifteen, the correct age for Thomas Joseph at that time. No daughter is listed, but it is possible that Annie Elizabeth had been sent to live with relatives after her father's death.[3]

On April 20, 1848, Ann's granddaughter and namesake, eighteen-year-old Annie Elizabeth Mattingly, married William Butler, and the 1850 census lists them living in Richmond, Virginia. A "Joseph" Mattingly, born in Virginia in June 1827, a printer, appears in the 1850 District of Columbia census living in Ward 2 of the city. Following the breach with the Carbery family, Thomas seems to have abandoned his use of his uncle the captain's name in favor of "Joseph." On November 18, 1853, Ann's grandson married Hannah Reeves, whose name also appears as Anna. Methodist ministers performed the marriages of both Annie Elizabeth and Thomas Joseph Mattingly. For the Catholic Carberys, a defection to Methodism alone might have been enough to cause a breach. We have seen that their mother, Harriet, was likely of mixed race. The marriages of both her children in the Methodist Church suggest she was perhaps also affiliated with this church.[4]

In 1850, Ann Mattingly was living at the home of her daughter, Susan, and her husband Richard Lay and their six children. In 1846, while Thomas Joseph and Annie Elizabeth, her grandchildren by her son, also lived in Washington, Ann Mattingly had made her last will and testament in her own hand. In it she writes that "after committing my Soul into the hand of Almighty God, and my body to the Earth," and after the payment of all her debts and funeral expenses, her property should be passed down to the family of Susan and Richard Lay. Nothing was left to her son John's children; her will does not mention them at all. Furthermore, Thomas Carbery, in contemplating distribution of his substantial estate, is equally severe toward Thomas Joseph and Annie Elizabeth. After portioning his large estate to his remaining sisters and chosen nieces and nephews, Carbery left the bulk of the estate, a large one worth about $250,000 at his death in 1863 (between $3.5 and $4.2 million today), to the St. Vincent's Orphan Asylum. Thomas and Annie, now themselves orphans, were not named as heirs.[5]

One of the Lay descendents told me he had long been aware that a breach had occurred between branches of the family a few generations before. Many family members knew there had been a "scandal" but did not know the details. Mrs. Clarke had labored for many years on the Mattingly genealogy until it seemed to her that John Baptist Carbery Mattingly would in fact, "yield to no one." There was an unusual silence about John in the historical record. The family theory had been that her mother's and grandfather's deeply olive complexions, despite their English, Irish, and

German ancestry, suggested that, far back, some racial mixing had occurred. Both Mrs. Clarke and descendents of Annie Elizabeth Mattingly
had wondered especially about a photo of one of Annie's daughters, which
showed a dark-skinned child with kinky hair. At my request, fair-skinned,
blue-eyed Mrs. Clarke, Mrs. Mattingly's great-great-great-granddaughter,
agreed to take a DNA test that revealed, among other things, that she is
11 percent "sub-Saharan African." In other words, she likely had an African ancestor. This test, in conjunction with a series of family photos in
the hands of descendents, reveals a source of the breach that goes beyond
marrying outside of the family religion. It appears that Harriet Doyle Mattingly was of mixed race. Most likely she was free, because John would not
have been permitted by law to marry a slave. Harriet's father, Martin Doyle,
moved to Washington near the canal, an area where Irish and black residents
mixed freely. We know little of Harriet's mother, except that she was living
in 1830 with Martin Doyle in a small frame house in Washington. That year,
while he was confined to the Washington jail for debt, Doyle requested release because his family was sick and he needed to help his wife with their
care. Since John and Harriet Mattingly also returned to Washington about
1830, it is possible that they were staying with the Doyles and that John was
sick, perhaps with the creeping paralysis. At least two doctors appear on
Doyle's list of creditors.[6]

The name Doyle appears on a Rootsweb list of "Melungeon sur-
names" associated with mixed-race groups of white, Native American, and
African ancestry. Some believe that the Melungeons are descended from
Portuguese, Spanish, Turkish, Jewish, and other Mediterranean peoples,
both free and slaves, connected to the settlement of Florida. Mixed-race
people in southern Maryland were known as the Wesorts. Depending on
which story you believe, the name Wesort has at least two possible origins.
One states that the Piscataway Native Americans described themselves as,
"we sorts of Mulattos, we sorts of Indian." The other anecdote about the
name's origins is more exclusionary, with the mixed-race group saying to
African Americans, "we sorts of people don't mix with you sorts of people."
While Harriet Doyle Mattingly's origins are shrouded, DNA evidence sheds

important light on the photographic evidence and suggests that Harriet was of mixed race.[7]

John and Harriet Mattingly's children, Thomas Joseph and Annie Elizabeth Mattingly, do not necessarily have identifiable African facial features such as olive skin and dark curly hair (see photos; Annie Elizabeth shown with an unknown young child, possibly Walter Joseph Ningard). Thomas Joseph bears a resemblance to his great-uncle, Captain Thomas Carbery (see photo). But in the next generation, the children of both Annie Elizabeth and Thomas Joseph have more distinctly sub-Saharan features (see photos of Rebecca Ningard Stout, Annie Elizabeth's daughter, and Harriet M. Mattingly, Martina Mattingly, and Joseph Carbery Mattingly, Thomas Joseph's two daughters and son—all Ann Mattingly's great-grandchildren). The photographic evidence that has remained in family archives suggests that the family breach may have resulted from John Mattingly's union with the multiracial Harriet Doyle.

In 1826, Mrs. Anne Royall, a famous traveler, published a book that reveals some of the attitudes of Americans toward miscegenation. During her 1824 trip through what is now West Virginia, the frontier country where John had fled with Harriet, Royall was shocked to encounter a Dutch family whose daughters had borne children fathered by men of African descent. Arriving in Alexandra, Virginia, Royall records her response to seeing men and women of mixed race in the public square:

> To one unaccustomed to see human nature in this guise, it excites feelings of horror and disgust. It has something in it so contrary to nature, something which seems never to have entered into her scheme, to see a man neither black nor white, with blue eyes, and a woolly head, has something in it at which the mind recoils. It appears that these people, instead of abolishing slavery, are gradually not only becoming slaves themselves, but changing color . . . But for a man in this free, and (as they say) enlightened country, to doom his own children, to a state (to say the least of it,) fraught with every species of human misery,

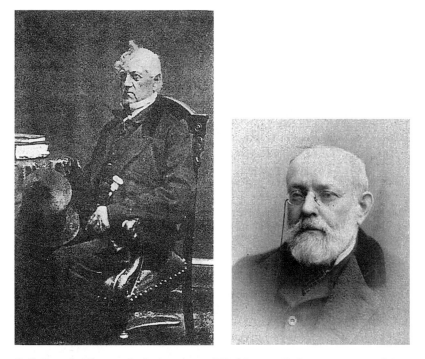

(*left*) Captain Thomas Carbery, mayor of Washington, D.C., 1822–1824, and Ann
Mattingly's brother, ca. 1850. Private collection. (*right*) Thomas Joseph Mattingly,
Ann Mattingly's grandson, who bears a resemblance to his great-uncle Captain
Thomas Carbery, ca. 1880–1890. Private collection.

we want no better evidence to prove, that such men must not
only be devoid of virtue, but guilty of the most indignant crime.[8]

Royall's response grew out of a culture based on a series of prohibitions
against racial mixing from the earliest days. That the codes were widely
ignored by slaveholders does not take away from their harshness. The Carberys of Washington owned domestic slaves, and it is not known whether
or not they would share Ann Royall's disgust at racial mixing.

Historian Letitia Woods Brown wrote that a 1691 Virginia law de-

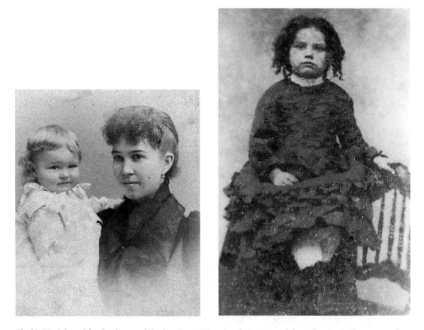

(*left*) Unidentified photo, likely Ann Mattingly's granddaughter and namesake, Annie Elizabeth Mattingly, with Walter Joseph Ningard, Ann Mattingly's great-grandson, ca. 1873. Private collection. (*right*) Rebecca Ningard Stout, born in 1867 to Annie Elizabeth Mattingly; great-granddaughter of Ann Mattingly. Private collection.

signed to prevent "abominable and spurious mixture" warned that any free white man or woman who married a Negro, mulatto, or Indian mate, bond or free, was within three months to be banished from the dominion forever. The infamous Code of 1715 not only forbade marriage between a white person and "any Negroe whatsoever or Molotto slave" but also penalized procreation between whites and Negroes. Brown notes that any white woman having a child by a Negro, slave or free, would herself become a servant for seven years. A white man who sired a child by a Negro woman, free or slave, and a free Negro who sired a child by a white woman were also, on conviction of the county court, sentenced to seven years' service.

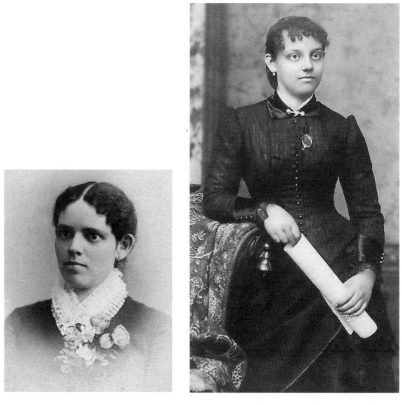

(*left*) Harriet M. Mattingly, daughter of Thomas Joseph Mattingly and Hannah Reeves; great-granddaughter of Ann Mattingly. Both Thomas Joseph and Annie Elizabeth named one of their daughters Harriet, supporting the likelihood that Ann Mattingly's son, John Baptist Carbery Mattingly, married Harriet Doyle. Private collection. (*right*) Martina M. Mattingly, daughter of Thomas Joseph Mattingly and Hannah Reeves; great-granddaughter of Ann Mattingly, ca. 1880. Private collection.

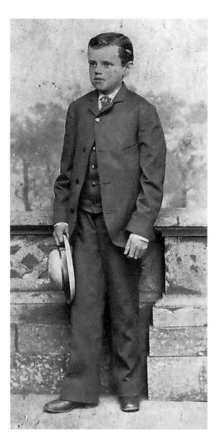

Joseph Carbery Mattingly, son
of Thomas Joseph Mattingly and
Hannah Reeves; great-grandson
of Ann Mattingly, ca. 1880.
Private collection.

Servants were expected to complete their current term and then serve another seven-year term. Any children of these unions would be forced to
serve until age thirty-one. Only in 1790 did the Maryland Assembly repeal
the acts imposing servitude of thirty-one years of the "issue of inordinate
copulations." The legislators felt it was "contrary to the dictates of humanity
and the principles of the Christian religion to inflict personal penalties on
children for the offenses of their parents," yet these children were nonethe-
less referred to as being of "peculiar descent."[9]

Royall's views about racial mixing reflect some of the predominant
attitudes in the country in the early nineteenth century, though the large

number of free black men and women living in the District of Columbia would mean that white and black people would have daily opportunities for interaction. According to historian Mary Beth Corrigan, free black men and women were the fastest growing population segment in the District, their numbers quintupling between 1800 and 1820 from about 780 to 4,050. In Washington City alone during this period, the free black population increased from 120 to nearly 1,700, and Georgetown's population swelled from 200 to 900. By 1830, free blacks outnumbered slaves in the District, with this trend continuing until the Civil War.[10]

Letitia Woods Brown analyzed the reasons for this significant increase, observing, "Racially mixed unions, though sometimes of minor interest elsewhere, were a significant factor in the District, in view of the large number of free mulattoes who resided there. Any attempt to account for the free Negro population of the District of Columbia would not be realistic without an analysis of this avenue of increase." The taboo against miscegenation was one of the strongest in the early American republic. The definition of a person's race depended on the idea of what kind of "blood" one carried, and the notion of the "one-drop rule" persisted well into the nineteenth century.[11]

Given the kind and depth of prejudice of the times expressed by Mrs. Royall, it seems reasonable to conclude that the Carbery family's unforgiving attitude toward John's children was based on his taboo interracial relationship with Harriet. Left out of both their grandmother Ann Mattingly's and Thomas Carbery's wills, Thomas Joseph and Annie Elizabeth joined with other relations to sue for a portion of the large estate of Captain Thomas Carbery, which he bequeathed to the St. Vincent Orphan Asylum after his death in 1863. With the suit of several relatives, the Sisters of Charity settled on a bequest of $15,000 (about $136,000 today). His will invalidated, Carbery was then considered as having died intestate, an ironic ending for a man who so thoroughly and carefully recorded his business doings throughout his life.

Not counting his other investments, Thomas Carbery's personal estate, including his "city residence" and a farm on Georgia Road, was worth more than $90,000. The extensive list of household items suggests a comfortable lifestyle in both town and country. The city residence on C and Seventeenth Streets included a sideboard, cut glass decanters, two large mahogany dining tables, and a horse carriage and wagon. At the fully furnished country house, forty acres of corn were "standing in the field," five acres of potatoes were growing, and the storehouse had an inventory that included two hundred gallons of vinegar. Thomas Carbery's executor, Richard Lay, husband of Susan Mattingly Lay, detailed the extensive property in several pages of legal briefs.[12]

Convoluted court proceedings of suits and countersuits stretched over a dozen years, beginning in 1863, with the deposition of witnesses to establish family relationships. Louisa Kearney testified that she had known Thomas Carbery intimately from childhood, nearly sixty years. She knew all his family and recalls hearing of a brother, "Jackey" (John Baptist Carbery), who died in 1803. Another witness, Eliza Barry, stated: "Mrs. Mattingly was the one of all the sisters that left any children. She left a daughter Mrs. Lay, and two children of a son John who died before Mrs. Mattingly. These two children of John, I had mostly lost sight of but I know one of them was named Joseph." Louisa Kearney also testified: "Mrs. Mattingly sister of Thomas Carbery died during the lifetime of Thomas Carbery. She survived her husband and she had two children, Mary Susan (now Mrs. Lay) now living and John who married and died [during] the lifetime of his mother leaving two children. I understand that both of these children are living and that the daughter was married. I know nothing of them. John Mattingly's wife is dead." These terse comments reflect the code of silence that surrounded all discussion of John Mattingly and John Baptist Carbery Mattingly.[13]

After the first round of lawsuits, the court ruled in 1866 that Thomas and Annie would receive $354.50 each (about $6,250 today). Susan Mattingly Lay received a substantial inheritance—the same amount as Thomas and Annie but also a quarter share of the bulk of the estate. Susan would die in 1871 at age sixty-five before the suit was fully settled. In 1865, what had become known as the "miracle house" built by Thomas Carbery on C and Seventeenth Streets was sold to William Galt for $4,500 (about $61,000 today), and another suit was filed regarding some income for Catharine Carbery, the mayor's sister, which he had decreed in his will. Thomas Joseph Mattingly, Ann's grandson, was called to testify. On March 9, 1866, a day before the forty-second anniversary of the Mattingly miracle, Thomas certified that he had attended one meeting about the distribution of the earlier will and that he had never read his uncle's will or heard it read. Clearly, there was minimal contact between Thomas Joseph Mattingly and the Carbery branches of the family. The battles over Thomas Carbery's estate lasted for fifteen years after his death, until 1878. Thomas and Annie were subsequently left out of the wills of other Carbery relatives: their great-aunts Catharine and Ruth Carbery and their aunt Susan Lay, who died after both Ann Mattingly and Thomas Carbery. Annie Elizabeth Mattingly Butler Rimby Ningard, whose death certificate lists her as "white," died in Baltimore in 1888 of consumption. She was about fifty-eight years old.[14]

When Thomas Joseph Mattingly died at his home in Oxon Hill, Maryland, January 23, 1908, at age eighty-one, his obituary described him as "one of the oldest and best known printers of Washington." He had been the publisher of the *Congressional Globe* and the journal of congressional events and debates until the government itself began disseminating the congressional record. Then, Thomas Joseph went to work for the U.S. government, retiring from the Government Printing Office after twenty-five years, having earned the affectionate nickname from his coworkers of "Uncle Joe" and a reputation for being an "authority on Congressional style." His wife, Hannah; two daughters, Harriet and Martina Mattingly; and one son, Joseph Carbery Mattingly, a lawyer, survived him. Two other children, Mary L. Mattingly Campbell and little Virgil Maxcy Mattingly, were not mentioned in the obituary. Though Thomas Joseph and his wife, Hannah Reeves, had been married in the Methodist Church, after the death of Virgil Mattingly in 1859, the family returned to Catholicism, baptizing their daughters in the Catholic St. Aloysius Church. Thomas Joseph was buried at St. Ignatius Catholic Church, Oxon Hill. It is striking that his youngest son Joseph was given the Carbery name despite the breach in the family relations. As a successful lawyer, Joseph Carbery Mattingly likely felt a close connection to the eminent Carbery family of Washington, D.C. With Joseph's success, the family seemed to have overcome the scandalous secret of John Baptist Carbery Mattingly's interracial marriage. On his father's death certificate, Thomas's race is listed as "white." But in the space where lawyer Joseph Carbery Mattingly was to write the names of Thomas's father and mother, he inexplicably wrote "unknown."[15]

Prince Hohenlohe's Final Years

After the Mattingly miracle of 1824, Prince Hohenlohe's reputation as a healer gained even more international prominence. During his extended leave from his position in Bamberg, the prince continued his attempts to cure sick people. Invalids traveled from as far away as England to see him. But the prince himself was in delicate health, having been susceptible to illness since he was a boy. When he traveled to Austria in 1842 to restore his fragile health, his fame as a miracle worker followed him, and again, sick people seeking his help thronged around him.

Several cures took place in France, both before and after the 1824 cure of Ann Mattingly and other North American cures. Perhaps the most famous French miracle is recounted in Albert Garreau's *L'Anneau d'Or: Spirituels de L'Allemagne Romantique* (The Golden Ring: Spiritual Stories of Romantic Germany), published in 1957. In 1828, Prince Hohenlohe met the well-known writer Honoré de Balzac in Paris. Balzac's mother had developed a strange illness: she could not eat raw fruits. If she did, her stomach became enormously bloated. According to Garreau, the prince simply asked her whether she believed in God: "Madame, croyez-vous en Dieu?" When she replied in the affirmative, she was instantly healed. Balzac enthusiastically wrote to his friend about his mother's healing, despite the fact that he was not always enthusiastic about religion.[16]

Hohenlohe's behavior toward Princess Mathilde von Schwarzenberg after he had so wonderfully cured her must have been something of a disappointment to her. On August 30, 1831, the prince asked her for a large loan to acquire a vineyard that was said to be profitable at 12 percent. His plan to pay the money back within three years with 5 percent interest was flawed.

Despite repeated reminders from the princess and her agents, the back-payment and interest remained delinquent, with the result that the princess petitioned the church hierarchy for intervention in 1848. Though Prince Hohenlohe offered excuses, the princess insisted on her receivables. She was given the last payment in 1848, after she had agreed to drop seventeen years' worth of interest.[17]

Prince Hohenlohe's promotion to bishop of Sardica, now Sofia, capital of Bulgaria, was finally granted in 1844. This was a title in name only, *in partibus infidelium,* meaning nonresidential, without a see, "in the lands of the unbelievers." His beloved mother did not see him reach this coveted goal, however, because she had died in 1836. The prince left Hungary in order to escape the revolutionary events and because of his poor health. But those who believed in his powers did not leave him alone. In Tyrol, Switzerland, the belief in Hohenlohe's power to work miracles was unusually strong. In his biography of the prince, Ludwig Sebastian numbers eighteen thousand visitors to whom Hohenlohe supposedly granted audience during his stay. By the end of September 1849, the severely ill prince, suffering from dropsy, a generalized edema usually associated with cardiac failure, returned to Vienna. One biographer reported on the deeply depressed Hohenlohe's last days: "His disease grew worse from day to day. His nerves grew so weak that he broke into loud tears for the least cause. He spent entire nights without sleep and if he napped for a few moments, sorrow caused him to awaken."[18]

The poet Heinrich Heine wrote a sonnet about Prince Hohenlohe called "Bamberg und Würzburg":

> In both these precincts flows the font of grace,
> A thousand miracles happen every day.
> See how the sick besiege in dense array
> The Prince who heals them all and right in place.
>
> He says: "Get up and walk!" Before your face
> The lame arise and briskly walk away.

"Look up!" he says, and "See now!" he may say,
Though born blind, they see in every case.

A youth comes forth, with dropsy sorely smitten:
"O wonder-worker, help my body's plight."
The Prince says, "Bless you! Go ye forth and write!"

In Bamberg and in Würzburg all get lyrical
And Gebhart's shop cries loudly: "It's a miracle!"
Nine plays already has that youth got written.[19]

Prince Alexander von Hohenlohe died on November 14, 1849, in Vös-
lau, close to Vienna, and was buried three days later next to his mother
in her family tomb of Baron Fries, as he had requested. Albert Garreau
described crowds of clergy and the faithful attending his funeral, including
the Prince of Schwarzenberg. Rev. Joseph Forster, pastor of Huttenheim in
Bavaria, continued to receive letters long after Prince Hohenlohe's death.
He answered them until his own death in 1875.[20]

Hohenlohe had many opponents as well as supporters, and some
remarkable results were attributed to him. Some credit Hohenlohe's healings with building greater participation in Catholic churches in Europe.
The prince was also a prolific author. He is said to have written more than
twenty editions of sermons before 1845 as well as several speeches, prayer
books, and prayers, though critics charge that many of these were ghost-
written. Popular portraits depict the prince as "God-chosen," especially
at the times of his miracle healings; he is often portrayed with a devotional
expression, his hands folded in prayer.

About his character, divided opinions remain. Some of his contemporaries in the clergy, such as J. M. Sailer, bishop of Regensburg, viewed him
as a holy and devoted person. Others, such as Professor Friedrich Brenner
of Bamberg, did not have a high opinion of him. That many people outside
the church had a strong antipathy toward the prince is demonstrated in the
attacks published in Western newspapers, including those in the United
States. As early as 1823, even supporters of his miracles sought to avoid the

"character question" about Prince Hohenlohe. Cassiodor Franz Joseph
Zenger created an imagined conversation between two friends about the
cures. At one point in the dialogue, the character named Benedict remarks
that Prince Hohenlohe is not being considered for sainthood and affirms
that no discussion is taking place about whether or not he is eligible: "We
do not even need to discuss his character. The topic of this conversation
is his action, the cures he performs." Zenger, however, supported the idea
of going forward with canonization on the basis of criteria outlined in the
Tridentine reforms.[21]

The Prince's biographer, Ludwig Sebastian, wrote that a very severe
judgment about Prince Hohenlohe came from Paul Johann von Feuerbach,
who claimed that he heard from the prince's brother, Prince Franz, that
Hohenlohe was a bad person who brought dishonor to the whole family:
"He is a juggler who does not pay his debts, he seduces girls, and he shows
off with his bad behavior among his friends." However, Sebastian stressed
that letters from Prince Franz do not validate von Feuerbach's accusations.
Still, these charges echo those made in many nineteenth-century publications, including *The Gentleman's Magazine,* that the prince was an atrocious
liar, frequently drunk, and lascivious. To his enemies, the prince was "an
itinerant Thaumaturgist, of blasted character." To admirers such as Sebastian, Hohenlohe seemed to lead a sound life, though he admits that some
negative accusations may have rung true.[22]

Sebastian believed that the prince was mostly a caring and loving person, who only wanted to cure sick people to help them out of their misery.
He adored his mother and was very affectionate toward her during her last
years. The prince was social and liked parties and celebrations. Despite all
these positive attributes, the prince also had negative ones, most notably his
inability to handle money and propensity to accumulate debts. Hohenlohe
was frequently accused of lying, especially about his miraculous cures,
since he promised healings that did not always come about. It is evident
that the prince craved recognition, seeking a prestigious appointment as a
bishop and literary fame. It will probably never be known whether he was
a philanderer.

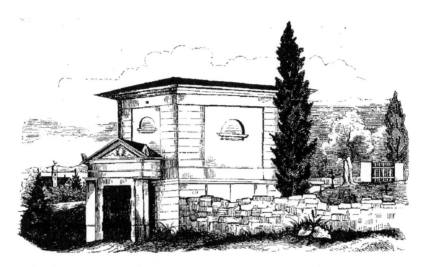

Sketch of Prince Alexander Hohenlohe's tomb from a book by Sebastian Brunner,
*Aus dem Nachlasse des Fürsten Alexander Hohenlohe, Bischof von Sardika, Gross-
probst von Grosswardein* (1851).

Ann Mattingly and Prince Hohenlohe held opposing views of their roles
in relation to miracle working and Catholicism, demonstrating some of
the tensions between lives lived inside and outside the Catholic Church
hierarchy. Mrs. Mattingly did not actively seek her cure but accepted what
was in store for her with a humble resignation to follow whatever path God
marked out for her. Despite the fame that engulfed her after the miracle, she
was an intensely private woman, a person who, unlike Prince Hohenlohe,
did not seek attention. But sadly, she was unable to choose her own path
during her second and third chances at life.

When Mrs. Mattingly first moved to the Capital City in 1805, Catholics had a strong foothold there. The city's voters elected her brother as its
mayor in 1822, and he served as a charter member and first vice president
of the Washington National Monument Society, formed in 1833. Because
of the influence of Catholic Maryland, Washington's culture was at first
very different from that of New England. But the enlightened tolerance of

the District of Columbia did not last. In the final two decades of Mrs. Mattingly's life, New England–style anti-Catholicism had gained new ascendancy on the national scene, reincarnated as the nativist, or Know-Nothing perspective. In March 1854, in a well-known anti-Catholic episode, a block of historic marble from Rome, a gift from Pope Pius IX for the Washington Monument, mysteriously disappeared. It seems likely that it was thrown into the Potomac River by members of the Know-Nothing Party. By the time of Ann Mattingly's death the following year, members of her Roman Catholic faith were regarded as threatening to American values and the American way of life.

Ann Mattingly's life spanned a period of tremendous change in the American Catholic Church. Until 1815, when Mrs. Mattingly moved into her brother Thomas Carbery's house in Washington, a single see, Baltimore, known as the Rome of the United States, governed the Catholic Church. The dominant Catholic consciousness was Anglo-American, a consciousness very much aligned with the mind-set of the nation's founders. By the time of Mrs. Mattingly's death in 1855, the American church was almost unrecognizable from the church of her birth. The flood of Irish immigrants that began in the 1820s permanently altered the homogenous Anglo-American character of the church, and it developed into an organization marked by internal ethnic rivalries. Historian Randall M. Miller notes that the sheer numbers of Catholic immigrants arriving in the second half of the nineteenth century "brought power and, in time, affluence to the Church, and . . . fostered a militancy and self-confidence . . . that in some ways discouraged the new Catholic population from assimilating into American culture and society." Hence, during the seven decades of Ann Mattingly's life, the American church moved away from assimilation to a marginalized status in the nation.[23]

Unlike the broader culture of the United States, which was in the throes of inventing the mythology of assimilation, the Catholic Church actively nurtured ethnic separation by founding parishes for various ethnic groups. This helped create in Catholics a sense of being a people apart from the mainstream. Nativism, of course, verified this perception and deepened the feelings of difference among Catholics. By the final decade of Mrs. Mattingly's life, the church had developed a self-protective strategy of vehemently defending Catholic values against attacks. The paradox of the ambivalent American Catholic identity is a theme that has been discussed by several scholars, including Edward Wakin, Joseph Scheuer, Andrew Greeley, and Jay Dolan.[24] In her youth, Ann Mattingly witnessed members of her family actively participate in building and governing the nation's capital; in her old age, she saw nativist violence single out Catholics as enemies within the nation. The deepening divide between North and South over the issue of slavery further fractured American Catholic identity. What became a personal breach over race in the Mattingly family exploded at the national level in a Civil War.

The Death of Ann Mattingly

Death is the ultimate betrayal of the soul by the body, and Ann Carbery Mattingly's final deathbed experience came on March 9, 1855, when she died peacefully at Norway, Thomas Carbery's three-hundred-acre farm where she had lived with her daughter and son-in-law, Susan and Richard Lay, and her grandchildren. The house where Ann died was located near present-day Walter Reed Hospital in Washington, D.C. It was burnt during the Civil War in 1864 during the Battle of Fort Stevens. Ann Mattingly did not live long enough to see the nation torn apart over slavery, although tensions over race destroyed her relationship with her son John. The enormous fame she had experienced thirty years before her death was not even noted in her obituary. The *National Intelligencer,* which had published so many controversial letters about the Mattingly miracle of 1824, gave this brief notice of Mrs. Mattingly's passing: "This amiable and pious lady, in a short but very severe illness, manifested a most perfect resignation to the will of God, and fortified by the holy sacraments of her church, met her death with calm and humble confidence."[25]

Nathaniel Hawthorne's daughter, Rose Hawthorne Lathrop, a convert to Catholicism, wrote a book, *A Story of Courage,* about miracles at the

Ann Mattingly's signature.

Visitation Monastery in Georgetown where Ann Mattingly spent so many months and experienced her second cure. Commenting on Rev. William Matthews' observation that Mrs. Mattingly had "suffered more than I had thought a mortal frame could endure," Lathrop meditates on the double meaning of the word *patient:* "Clearly, she was a 'patient' in the full sense of the word; a sufferer, yet resigned. Even indifferentists, and those who have no very active belief, agree that to be 'patient' means not merely to suffer, but to do so without complaint. The faithful hold the same view; but in addition, they look upon true suffering as a duty borne for God." Lathrop also quotes from a letter written by Ann's sister Catharine about the closing of "Miracle Ann's" life: "I remember most distinctly that a sister . . . and Carbery, eldest son of Mr. Richard Lay, upon going to the room where Mrs. Mattingly died, and which had been locked, with all the fetid air from confinement, the windows being closed during the entire sickness, and also from bedclothes soiled to an extreme, were amazed at the sweet odor of the room, and called myself and other members of the family to come; and we all wondered at such sweetness from such a mass of impurity."[26]

During the week that Mrs. Mattingly died, Washington again blossomed with the loveliness of March. The wonder of the city's spring flowers, especially the delicate cherry blossoms, can evoke for us the ebb and flow of human life in the nation's capital. Their fragrance can remind us of lives that merit commemoration in marble, but also of those uncounted Americans whose stories have much to teach us. Mrs. Mattingly had lived an exceptionally long life for the nineteenth century, during which the average life expectancy was only thirty-five to forty-five years. Had she died in March 1824, during her first deathbed experience at age thirty-nine, she would have lived out an ordinary lifespan for a woman of her day. But, as we have seen, her life did not run the usual course.

The day after she died, March 10, she was buried in St. Patrick's cemetery. Her funeral took place exactly thirty-one years after the miraculous cure that had snatched her from death. When Ann's daughter, Susan Mattingly Lay, died in 1871, and the cemetery at St. Patrick's was closing, the family purchased a burial plot at nearby Mount Olivet Cemetery. The remains of Thomas, Mary, Ruth, and Catharine Carbery, along with Ann Carbery Mattingly, were moved there. It is not known where John Mattingly or John Baptist Carbery Mattingly were laid to rest. If they had originally been interred at St. Patrick's, they were not moved with the others in 1871. Bodies and coffins continued to be found on the site of the old cemetery for years afterward. In 1951, someone, probably Joseph Carbery Mattingly, placed a stone monument for the family at Mount Olivet Cemetery. Ann's stone reads:

> Ann Carbery Mattingly
> Beloved Wife of John Mattingly
> March 17, 1784
> March 10, 1855

With the placement of this stone, the tragic dissolution of a marriage and the breaking apart of a family were reduced, as monuments have a way of doing, to chiseled shorthand for a much richer story.

In 1901, the Daughters of the American Revolution purchased the Carbery house with the intent of tearing it down; from the look of contemporary photos, it had fallen into disrepair. A watercolor by an unknown artist romanticizes the lonely dwelling a bit, and the house looks as though it has sad secrets to keep, and very possibly the ghost of Foggy Bottom to haunt it. It was razed in 1903, five years before the death of Ann's eldest grandson, Thomas Joseph Mattingly. The story of the Mattingly miracle is threaded through with questions of the porous border that separates doubt and belief. Shakespeare, C. S. Lewis, and many others through the ages have pondered the question of whether or not the finger of God can

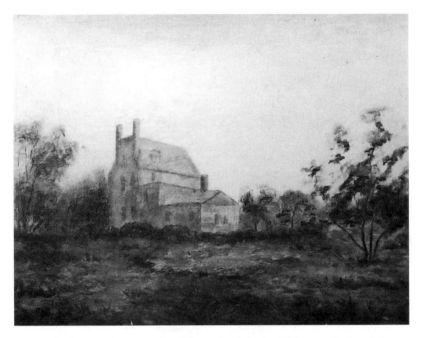

Watercolor by an unknown artist of the "miracle house," Thomas Carbery's house in Washington, D.C. Collection of Georgetown Visitation Monastery Archives.

reach out and touch us here on earth. Like C. S. Lewis, Rose Hawthorne Lathrop truly believed that miracles abound in this world. Sometimes, she says, they are remembered, and sometimes forgotten. The life of Ann Mattingly, touched with tragedy and special grace, joy and sorrow, and many thankfully unremarkable days, is, finally, not all that different from our own.

Cessit

Carbery-Mattingly Family Tree

John Baptist Carbery (born before 1647–1713)
|
John Baptist Carbery (1660–before 1729)
|
John Baptist Carbery (ca. 1702–before 1794)
|
Thomas Carbery (ca. 1745–1812); m. Mary Asenath Simmons
(ca. 1757–1819)
|

    Mary Carbery, Carmelite (1775–1858)

    John Baptist "Jackey" Carbery (1777–1803)

    Martha Carbery Catalano (1779–1857)

    Ruth Carbery (1780–1869)

    Ann Carbery Mattingly (1784–1855) (see below)

    Joseph Carbery, Jesuit (1786–1849)

    Catharine (1789–1880)

    Thomas (1791–1863)

    James (1793–1851)

    Lewis (1795–1860)

    Ignatius Henry (1797–1799)

**Ann Carbery; m. John Mattingly (see below), 1803, St. Mary's
County, Maryland**
|
Mary Susan Mattingly (1806–1871); m. Richard Lay, 1832
|

    Seven children: Anna Maria Lay Hook, Joseph Carbery Lay,
    Richard Gregory Lay, Thomas Wolcott Lay, Theodore Albert
    Lay, Albert H. Lay, William Matthews Lay

|

John Baptist Carbery Mattingly (1809–1839); m. Harriet Doyle, ca. 1827
|
    Thomas Joseph Mattingly (1827–1908); m. Hannah M. Reeves, 1853
    |
        Virgil Maxcy Mattingly (1854–1859)
        Harriet M. Mattingly (1857–1932)
        Mary Lillian Mattingly (1861–1894)
        Martina Mattingly (1866–1954)
        Joseph Carbery Mattingly (1871–1948)
        |
    Annie Elizabeth Mattingly Butler Rimby Ningard (ca. 1830–1888)
    |
        James Butler (1849–?)
        William H. Rimby (1856–1878)
        Harriet (Hattie) Rimby (1858–?)
        Jacob Gregory Rimby (1862–1864)
        Annie Rebecca Ningard Stout (1867–1943)
        Walter Joseph Ningard (1870–1938)
        |
    John Mattingly (ca. 1832–1833)

Mattinglys

Thomas Mattingly (ca. 1630–1664)
|
Cezar Mattingly (1654–ca. 1720)
|
John Mattingly (ca. 1685–ca. 1744)
|
John Baptist Mattingly (1715–1755)
|
James Barton Mattingly (1743–1812); m. Mildred Nevitt (17?–before 1813)
|
John Mattingly (17?–1822)

Notes

Prologue

1. This imagined scene is loosely based on a sketch of historical fiction by Marie Lomas, "Miracle House," undated photocopy, private collection.

2. C. S. Lewis, *Miracles: A Preliminary Study* (1947; repr. New York: Harper-Collins, 2001), 2. The Christian conception of miracles, according to *Easton's 1897 Bible Dictionary* (http://dictionary.reference.com/browse/miracle, accessed August 4, 2010), is strongly influenced by accounts in the New Testament, where four Greek words, *semeion, terata, dunameis,* and *erga,* are used to describe the phenomenon. S*emeion,* or "sign," appears in the gospels of Matthew, Mark, Luke, and John. These signs are viewed as "evidence of a divine commission; an attestation of a divine message" and as "a token of the presence and working of God; the seal of a higher power." *Terata,* meaning "wonders," appears in Acts, referring to "wonder-causing events . . . portents . . . [that produce] astonishment in the beholder." The scribe of Acts also uses the word *dunameis,* or "mighty works" or "works of superhuman power," to connote a "new and higher power"; the word is also found in Romans and Thessalonians. Finally, the apostle John uses the word *erga,* meaning "the works of Him who is 'wonderful in working.'" Many Christians consider the stories of Jesus' miraculous cure of lepers, the blind, and the deaf and of raising the dead to be evidence of both his divinity and the operation of a supernatural hand in the world.

Chapter 1. Introduction

1. The death room scene is constructed from draft documents in the hand of Stephen Dubuisson, "Mrs. Mattingly's Affair," Maryland Province Archives (hereafter MPA), 14, 1, Georgetown University Library, Special Collections Division, Washington, DC, and material from William Matthews, *A Collection of Affidavits and Certificates, Relative to the Wonderful Cure of Mrs. Ann Mattingly Which Took Place in the City of Washington, D.C. on the Tenth of March, 1824* (Washington, DC, 1824). The quotation is from Matthews, 9.

2. Matthews, *Collection of Affidavits and Certificates,* 9.

3. "Hohenlohe, Alexander Leopold, prince of," *Encyclopedia Americana: A Popu-*

lar Dictionary of Arts, Sciences, Literature, History, Politics, and Biography, ed. Francis Leiber, vol. VI (1838), 386–387.

4. Letter from Kate Gideon Colt, February 2, 1907, private collection.

5. Dubuisson fragment, MPA, 13, 16.

6. Joseph P. Chinnici, O.F.M., *Living Stones: The History and Structure of Catholic Spiritual Life in the United States,* 2nd ed. (Maryknoll, NY: Orbis, 1996), 24–25.

7. Quoted in *An Examination of a Protestant's Objections to the Popish Miracle Lately Wrought in America* (London, 1824), 7.

8. Chrysostom, "Miraculous Cures," *Washington Theological Repertory,* April 1, 1824, 327; letter from Mary Apollonia Digges to Dubuisson, Georgetown, May 5, 1831, MPA, 210, quoted in Robert Emmett Curran, "'The Finger of God Is Here': The Advent of the Miraculous in the Nineteenth-Century American Catholic Community," *Catholic Historical Review* 73, no. 1 (1987): 41–61, 54n; *Diary of Brother Joseph Mobberly,* vol. IV, November 5, 1824, quoting *National Journal,* October 25, 1824.

9. Heather D. Curtis, *Faith in the Great Physician: Suffering and Divine Healing in American Culture, 1860–1900* (Baltimore, MD: Johns Hopkins University Press, 2007), 201.

10. Ibid., 16; Barbara Welter, "The Cult of True Womanhood: 1820–1860," *American Quarterly* 18, no. 2, part I (summer 1966), 151–174.

11. Curtis, *Faith in the Great Physician,* 17; Carolyn Walker Bynum, *Holy Feast and Holy Fast: The Religious Significance of Food to Medieval Women* (Berkeley: University of California Press, 1987), 209. The examples of Ebner and the connection to Bynum's work are also in Curtis, *Faith in the Great Physician,* 38. See also the work of Paula Kane on the topic of female spirituality linked to suffering, for example, "'She Offered Herself Up': The Victim Soul and Victim Spirituality in Catholicism," *Church History* 71, no. 1 (March 2002).

12. There is not a large body of scholarship on the history of miracles in the United States. Most texts on miracle history are devoted to the foundation of the Church of Rome and the medieval period. Scholars focusing on the miraculous during the nineteenth century study primarily Catholic European countries such as France, Italy, and Spain. Many books and articles allude briefly to Prince Hohenlohe's wonderworking in the nineteenth century, but he is allotted just a few pages in each of them. Thomas Kselman's *Miracles and Prophecies in Nineteenth-Century France* (New Brunswick, NJ: Rutgers University Press, 1983), examines Prince Hohenlohe's cures in France as reported in the transatlantic journal *L'Ami de Religion,* which Kselman describes as "the

most widely distributed religious journal of the Restoration, which had close ties with the French hierarchy" (23). Kselman includes a few pages on Prince Hohenlohe, noting Hohenlohe's transition from using the practices of lay healer to prescribing novenas and Masses, which the historian calls an example of the process of "absorption and adaptation of traditional ritual by orthodox religion." Kselman's main interest, then, is in the evolution of the prince's healing methods as an example of the priest's appropriation of traditional healing methods. His study of miracles is influenced by the work of Charles Guignebert in 1935, whose *Jesus* (trans. S. H. Hooke, New York: University Books, 1956) points out the impossibility of "the historian getting back to the exact fact which is described as miraculous" (191) and concentrates on the belief system that transcribed and promoted the miraculous event. Ann Taves, in *The Household of Faith: Roman Catholic Devotions in Mid-Nineteenth-Century America* (Notre Dame, IN: University of Notre Dame Press, 1986), also makes note of the Mattingly miracle, discussing it as an example of a sacred action that connected the American Catholic Church with sources of sacred power originating in Europe (57–58). Again, Taves's main interest is not in the prince himself, but in the curious aberration of the Mattingly miracle in American culture. A decade later, *Miracles and the Modern Religious Imagination* (New Haven, CT: Yale University Press, 1996), by Robert Bruce Mullin, devotes three pages to the Mattingly miracle. Mullin analyzes the compilation of affidavits attesting to the miracle by Bishop John England as an example of "the hoary Protestant Common Sense tradition being turned upon itself" (118). Mullin focuses on the varying responses of Protestants and Catholics in terms of their faith in miraculous occurrences. Additional books that discuss the Mattingly miracle include Robert Emmett Curran, *The Bicentennial History of Georgetown University, from Academy to University, 1789–1889,* vol. 1 (Washington, DC: Georgetown University Press, 1993); Morris J. MacGregor, *A Parish for the Federal City: St. Patrick's in Washington, 1794–1994* (Washington, DC: Catholic University of America Press, 1994); and William W. Warner, *At Peace with All Their Neighbors: Catholics and Catholicism in the National Capital, 1787–1860* (Washington, DC: Georgetown University Press, 1994). In 1870, Georgetown-born Anna H. Dorsey (1815–1896) published a novel called *The Old Gray Rosary* in which she retells the story of the Mattingly miracle. Though Dorsey was about nine years old at the time of the miracle, her conversion to Catholicism came after her marriage in 1837. In addition to these few books that refer briefly to the Mattingly miracles, one unpublished dissertation and a few essays look at the Mattingly cures in more detail. A

1938 master's thesis by Catholic University of America Benedictine Sister M. Mirella Burns, O.S.B., *An American Phase in the Life of Prince Alexander von Hohenlohe (1794–1849)*, is the lengthiest treatment of the events, at ninety-three pages, drawn largely from secondary sources. Robert Emmett Curran's essay "'The Finger of God Is Here'" has been the most comprehensive study of the Mattingly miracle available. See also Nancy Lusignan Schultz, "Miraculous Meddlings: Prince Hohenlohe's Transatlantic Intercessions in Washington, D.C. and in Charlestown, Massachusetts, 1824–1827," *U.S. Catholic Historian* 20, no. 1 (winter 2002): 1–19, and "Wunderbar," *Boston College Magazine* (spring 2002), 9–10. A more recent article by Laurence M. Geary, "Prince Hohen-lohe, Signor Pastorini and Miraculous Healing in Early Nineteenth-Century Ireland," in *Medicine, Disease and the State in Ireland, 1650–1940*, ed. Greta Jones and Elizabeth Malcolm (Cork, Ireland: Cork University Press, 1999), illuminates Hohenlohe's Irish cures during the summer of 1823. I am grateful to Claire Connelly for bringing this article to my attention. See also Marie Pagliarini's article, "'And the Word Was Made Flesh': Divining the Female Body in Nineteenth-Century American and Catholic Culture," *Religion and American Culture* 17, no. 2 (summer 2007): 213–245. In general, interest in the Mattingly miracle and in Prince Hohenlohe waned considerably beginning in the late nineteenth century. Several German studies of Prince Hohenlohe treat his European cures and were consulted as resources for this book.

Chapter 2. The Prince and the Princess

1. Mathilde's brother Felix, born in 1800, would later serve as prime minister of Austria from 1848 to 1852; a younger brother, Friedrich, born in 1809, would be ordained archbishop of Prague. Their father, Joseph von Schwarzenberg (1769–1833), is credited with finishing a navigational canal that facilitated wood transport from Bohemian forests to Vienna. He founded both a school of for-estry and the Schwarzenberg Economic Institute in Český Krumlov, where generations of nobles would be educated. The von Schwarzenbergs had nine children, one of whom died in infancy. The details of Mathilde's childhood are drawn from Ludwig Sebastian, *Fürst Alexander von Hohenlohe-Schillingsfürst, 1794 bis 1849 und Seine Gebets-Heilungen* (Bamberg, 1918).

2. Though some sources say Ambassador Schwarzenberg arranged the nuptials, most scholars believe that Prince Klemens von Metternich was responsible for the marriage agreement. Napoleon, in addition to wanting an heir, desired to strengthen his legitimacy as ruler by a marriage alliance with some of Europe's

old-line noble families. I am grateful to Annette Chapman-Adisho for her advice on sections relating to Napoleon.

3. The descriptions of the building and the ball are based on Imbert de Saint-Amand, *The Happy Days of the Empress Marie Louise,* trans. Thomas Sergeant Perry (New York: Charles Scribner's Sons, 1890), 224–235.

4. The narrative of the fire is based on Saint-Amand, *Happy Days,* and on Louis François Lejeune, N. d'Anvers, and John Frederick Maurice, *Memoirs of Baron Lejeune: Aide-de-camp to Marshals Berthier, Davout, and Oudinot,* vol. II, trans. Mrs. Arthur Bell (New York: Longmans, Green, 1897), 32–36 ("rapidity of lightning," 33).

5. Ibid., 33–34.

6. Ibid., 34.

7. Ibid., 35; *Moniteur,* July 3, 1810, quoted in Saint-Amand, *Happy Days,* 231.

8. Napoleon quoted in Louis Constant Wairy, *Recollections of the Private Life of Napoleon Bonaparte,* vol. II, XXVII (London, 1811), http://www.classicreader .com/book/3755/60 (accessed August 7, 2010). Having witnessed firsthand the helplessness of the volunteer firefighters in the face of this fire, Napoleon reorganized the service and converted it into a branch of the military. The embassy fire, then, was the catalyst for the foundation of Paris's first professional corps of firefighters, the Paris Fire Brigade. Felicia Dorothea Browne Hemans, *Records of Woman: With Other Poems,* ed. Paula R. Feldman (Lexington: University Press of Kentucky, 1999), 63–67.

9. Stephan Baron von Koskull, *Wunderglaube und Medizin, Die religiösen Heilungsversuche des Fürsten Alexander von Hohenlohe in Franken, 1821–1822* (Bamberg: Historischer Verein Bamberg Für die Pflege der Geschichte des ehemaligen Fürstbistums Bamberg, 22. Beiheft, 1988), 8, my translation.

10. Marie Pauline died two days after her fourth wedding anniversary. The summary of Mathilde's cures is based on Christian August Fischer, *Die merkwürdige Heilungsgeschichte der Fürstin Mathilde v. Schwarzenberg* (Berlin, 1821).

11. Sigmund Lahner, *"Der Wunderdoktor": Martin Michel von Unterwittighausen im Bad. Frankenland (1759–1824),* Oberwittighausen, Kreis Tauberbischofsheim, Druck: Wilhelm Beutel, Karlsruhe, 2, Auflage (collection of Universitätsbibliothek Eichstätt), 11.

12. Sebastian, *Fürst Alexander von Hohenlohe-Schillingsfürst,* 34. On Gassner, see H. C. Erik Midelfort, *Exorcism and Enlightenment: Johann Joseph Gassner and the Demons of Eighteenth-Century Germany* (New Haven, CT: Yale University Press, 2005). On Martin Michel, see Lahner, *"Der Wunderdoktor."*

13. Sebastian, *Fürst Alexander von Hohenlohe-Schillingsfürst,* 34.

14. Lahner, *"Der Wunderdoktor,"* 8.

15. Ibid., 9.

16. M. Mirella Burns, O.S.B., *An American Phase in the Life of Prince Alexander von Hohenlohe, 1794–1849* (M.A. Thesis, Catholic University of America, 1938), 9. I am grateful to Christopher Kauffman for his assistance in helping me obtain this source. The detail about Michel massaging the prince's neck and throat is in Herbert Thurston, "The Healing Hand: Prince von Hohenlohe," *Month,* 160, no. CLX (1932): 323–333.

17. Alexander, Prince de Hohenlohe, *Mémoires et expériences dans la vie sacerdotale et dans le commerce avec le monde, recueillis dans les années 1815–1834* (Paris, 1836), 51–56.

18. Description of the events of Princess Mathilde's cure is from Fischer, *Die merkwürdige Heilungsgeschichte,* 17–26, 31–32, my translation.

19. Ibid., 28, my translation.

20. Ibid., 50–52, my translation. The translation of Goethe (from *Wilhelm Meister's Apprenticeship and Travels,* Book I, Chap. 13) is Thomas Carlyle's.

21. Lahner, *"Der Wunderdoktor,"* 18, 27.

22. P. Beda Bastgen, *Der Heilige Stuhl und Alexander v. Hohenlohe-Schillingsfürst: Nach Akten des Vatikanischen Geheimarchivs* (1938), 40–41; Fischer, *Die merkwürdige Heilungsgeschichte,* 57–58, my translation; Lahner, *"Der Wunderdoktor,"* 19–20; Sebastian, *Fürst Alexander von Hohenlohe-Schillingsfürst,* 35; Thurston, "The Healing Hand," 328.

23. Fischer, *Die merkwürdige Heilungsgeschichte,* 57–58, my translation; Lahner, *"Der Wunderdoktor,"* 19–20; Sebastian, *Fürst Alexander von Hohenlohe-Schillingsfürst,* 35; Thurston, "The Healing Hand," 328; Henricus Tomas, *Aanspraak ter gelegenheid van een' plegtigen dankdienst: Opgedragen den 2 Sept: 1824 in de R. K. Kerk van den H. Thomas van Aquinen te Haarlem. Amsterdam* (C. C. Schievenbus, 1824). Special thanks to Geertje E. Wiersma for her assistance with the translation of the Dutch. On Michel, see Lahner, *"Der Wunderdoktor,"* 63–64.

24. Fischer, *Die merkwürdige Heilungsgeschichte,* 67–70, my translation.

Chapter 3. From St. Mary's County, Southern Maryland, to the Federal City

1. This retelling of the legend of Moll Dyer is a synthesis of two sources: Ed Okonowicz, *Haunted Maryland: Ghosts and Strange Phenomena of the Old Line State* (Mechanicsburg, PA: Stackpole, 2007), 95–97, and Jason Babcock,

"Witch or Not, Moll Dyer Legend Lives On," SoMdNews.com, October 30, 2009, http://www.somdnews.com/stories/10302009/entetop175334_32180 .shtml (accessed August 8, 2010). On October 14, 1972, the 875-pound boulder said to feature the handprint was moved to the front of the St. Mary's County Historical Society in Leonardtown, Maryland. The legend of Moll Dyer inspired the popular film *The Blair Witch Project* (1999).

2. From Revolution to Reconstruction, "The Maryland Toleration Act (1649)," http://www.let.rug.nl/~usa/D/1601-1650/maryland/mta.htm (accessed August 8, 2010).

3. Manuel Borutta, "Enemies at the Gate: The Moabit *Klostersturm* and the *Kulturkampf:* Germany," in *Culture Wars: Secular-Catholic Conflict in Nineteenth-Century Europe,* ed. Christopher Clark and Wolfram Kaiser (Cambridge: Cambridge University Press, 2003), 227–254. As Borutta observes, "Protestantism was characterized by the hegemony of liberal interest that pressed for the breakthrough into modernity—the ultramontanism of Catholicism entailed the marginalization and in some cases secession of pro-modern forces. In the *Syllabus errorum* of 1864—the papacy itself defined Catholicism as the antithesis of modernity" (227–228).

4. Edith Harden Ridout, "Peggy Stewart Tea Party Chapter," *American Monthly Magazine: Daughters of the American Revolution Magazine 33* (July–December 1908), 456–461.

5. The reconstruction of John Baptist Carbery's voyage to America is based on the narrative of Rose L. Martin, *The Story of Elizabeth: Our Country's First Nun* (New York: Twin Circle, 1968), 6. I am grateful to John Gottscho for bringing this narrative to my attention. Allen C. Clark's essay, "Mayors of the Corporation of Washington," in *Records of the Columbia Historical Society of Washington, D.C.,* published by Columbia Historical Society, 19 (1916): 62, states that John Baptist Carbery sailed from Ireland to Boston in about 1730 but does not offer evidence for the claim.

6. Margaret K. Fresco, *Marriages and Deaths in St. Mary's County* (Leonardtown, MD: St. Mary's County Historical Society, 1982), 49. See also Martin, *Story of Elizabeth,* 6; Vernon L. Skinner Jr., *Abstracts of the Testamentary Proceedings of the Prerogative Court of Maryland 7,* 1693–1697, 14A:10 and 15A:14.

7. Martin, *Story of Elizabeth,* 7; Clark, "Mayors of the Corporation," 62.

8. Suburban Emergency Management Project, "Ben Franklin's Exceptional View that Volcanic Eruptions Affect Climate," http://www.semp.us/publications/ biot_reader.php?BiotID=222 (accessed August 8, 2010).

9. John Gilmary Shea, *Life and Times of the Most Rev. John Carroll, Bishop and*

First Archbishop of Baltimore, Embracing the History of the Catholic Church in the United States, 1763–1815 (1888), 257–259.

10. Chinnici, *Living Stones,* 30, 7, 8–11.

11. Shea, *John Carroll,* 259; the saying is from Martin, *Story of Elizabeth,* 23.

12. This description of Ann's childhood is based on Martin's account of the early days of Ann's aunt, Elizabeth Carbery; Martin, *Story of Elizabeth,* 9–11.

13. Ibid., 11; the description of Ann's disposition is from notes by Stephen Dubuisson, fragment, MPA, 13, 16.

14. Details about the weather are from John Tessier, *Diary of Rev. John Tessier,* Archives of the Archdiocese of Baltimore (hereafter AAB), RG1, Box 9A, 1796–1835; other details are from a private family collection.

15. Shea, *John Carroll,* 399.

16. James Barton Mattingly (1743–1812) was son of John, son of John, son of Cezar, son of Thomas, and married Mildred Nevitt. See Timothy J. O'Rourke, *Catholic Families of Southern Maryland* (Baltimore, MD: Genealogical Publishing Company, repr. 2001); the "Register of Baptisms and Marriages, Congregations of St. Francis Xavier and St. Inigoes, St. Mary's County, Maryland," *1800 Federal Census,* St. Mary's County, Maryland, shows, for October 30, 1767, "Mattingly of Barton, Sp: Joseph & Rachel Nivet, bro & sister of Barton's wife, p. 18." and for March 31, 1777, "Thomas Mattingly of Bartholomew and Mildred, SP: Joseph and Mary Nevitt." At his death in 1813, James Barton Mattingly's entire estate was valued at $146.23, approximately $2,000 in today's currency.

17. Newtown Account Book, MPA, 452, 171 C.

18. Clark, "Mayors of the Corporation," 63, gives the death date of John Baptist Carbery as October 5, 1803; John B. Carbery's obituary appears in the *Republican Advocate,* Fredericktown, Maryland, October 7, 1803, 2.

19. Regina Combs Hammett, *History of St. Mary's County* (Ridge, MD: R. C. Hammett, 1977), lists Ann's father Thomas as "millowner," Upper Newton, and leaving for Washington, D.C., "after 180?," 86; Aleck Loker, *A Most Convenient Place: Leonardtown, MD (1650–1950)* (Leonardtown, MD: Commissioners of Leonardtown and Solitude Press, 2001), 38.

20. Loker, *Convenient Place,* 41.

21. Clark, "Mayors of the Corporation," 62; Samuel C. Busey, *Pictures of the City of Washington in the Past* (Washington, DC: Wm. Ballantyne & Sons, 1898), 235.

22. Thomas Moore, "Epistle VII to Thomas Hume, ESQ. M.D. from the City of Washington," in *The Poetical Works of Thomas Moore Including His Melodies, Ballads, etc: Complete in One Volume* (Paris: A. & W. Galignani, 1829), 101.

23. Busey, *City of Washington,* 159–163.
24. D.C. Historic Preservation Office, "Capital Hill Historic District," http://www
    .planning.dc.gov/planning/lib/planning/preservation/brochures/capitolhill
    broch.hi.pdf (accessed August 9, 2010), 6. See also Thomas B. Grooms and
    Taylor J. Lednum, *The Majesty of Capitol Hill* (Gretna, LA: Pelican, 2005),
    29–31; Madison Davis, "The Navy Yard Section during the Life of William
    Ryland," *Records of the Columbia Historical Society* 4 (1901): 220–221. The
    house was built for Thomas Carbery by Hugh Densley, a master plasterer who
    was one of the city's earliest craftsmen. Detail about the weather on September
    20, 1806, is from Tessier, *Diary.*
25. Weather detail from Tessier, *Diary.* Special thanks to Emerson "Tad" Baker,
    who helped me with the knotty problem of figuring out why John Mattingly is
    not named in the distribution though he appears in the will. Tad developed
    the following spreadsheet from the distribution.

> *The account of James Barton Mattingly, June 4, 1813*

Estate Accounted for	194.005	
Payments and Disbursements allowed	47.77	
Remainder and Distributable	146.235	
Distributions as follows, to wit:		
The Widow's thirds	48.745	85.3
Daughter Pann, one-eighth part	12.19	
Son Stephen	14.2166	
Daughter Ann	14.2166	
Son Thomas	14.2166	
Grandson Joseph Johnson	14.2166	
Granddaughter Mary Johnson	14.2166	
Given Total	146.235	
Actual Total	132.018	
Missing Sum (one-sixth of remainder)	14.217	

The amount $14.2166 equals one-sixth of the $85.30 remaining in the estate
after the distributions to the widow and daughter Pann. Since only five heirs
are named and the value of one share is missing, it can be safely assumed that
John Mattingly was omitted by clerical error but that he did actually inherit

$14.2166 from his father's estate. Series C1594, Estate Papers, Maryland State Archives, Annapolis.

26. "Record Group 94: Records of the Adjutant General's Office," *Compiled Military Service Records of Volunteer Soldiers Who Served in the War of 1812,* John Mattingly, Major King's Detachment, District of Columbia Militia, National Archives and Records Administration, Washington, DC.

27. Christian Hines, *Early Recollections of Washington City* (Washington, DC, 1866), 80.

28. Ibid., 81–82.

29. John McGowan v. John Mattingly (debt of $1,078.72), Record Group 21, Records of the District Court of the United States, District of Columbia, Entry 6, Case Papers Containing Appearances, Imparlances, etc., 1802–1863, December Term 1818, Civil Trials No. 444, National Archives and Records Administration, Washington, DC; author's communication with Linda Reno, June 13, 2007: "References to Joseph Nevitt in District records link him or them to other families who all kept inns and taverns. Joseph Nevitt Jr. married Barbara Willet, of a family that had inns on River Road and elsewhere. John Tennally (whose name survives in Tenleytown) kept an inn; when his sister and heir Sarah wrote her will, Joseph Nevitt Jr. was her executor, and Barbara Nevitt her witness. Sarah Tennally's house and furniture went to the daughter of Theophilus Robey, an innkeeper with whom Joseph Nevitt owned land in partnership. A Joseph Nevitt was one of the executors of Robey's will. Henry Riszner also had an inn in Tenleytown, but in 1816 he sold it and bought one of Joseph Nevitt's houses in this neighborhood."

30. Peter J. Smith, "The Mattingly Gene: A Crippling Disease in 11 Generations of a Maryland Family Offers Clues to a Medical Mystery," *Life Magazine* (fall 1998), 39–48. See also "Mattingly Family Featured in Life Magazine," *ALS Newsletter,* http://www.als-mda.org/Publications/als/als3_4.html#mattingly; Margaret Wahl, "Gene Mapped for Early-Onset Slowly Progressive Form of ALS," *MDA News,* March 13, 1998, http://www.mda.org/news/980313alsc9.html, and Wahl, "Gene Found in Early-Onset ALS," *MDA/ALS Newsmagazine* 9, no. 5 (May 2004), http://www.als-mda.org/publications/als/als9_5.html (all accessed August 10, 2010). Research studies on the disease include P. F. Chance et al., "Linkage of the Gene for an Autosomal Dominant Form of Juvenile Amyotrophic Lateral Sclerosis to Chromosome 9q34," *American Journal of Human Genetics* 62 (1998): 633–640, and Y. Z. Chen et al., "DNA/RNA Helicase Gene Mutations in a Form of Juvenile Amyotrophic Lateral Sclerosis (ALS4)," *American Journal of Human Genetics* 74, no. 6 (June 2004): 1128–1135.

31. For information on Carbery Wharf, see James M. Goode, *Capital Losses: A Cultural History of Washington's Destroyed Buildings* (Washington, DC: Smithsonian Institution, 2003), 15.

32. John McGowan v. John Mattingly debt.

33. Goode, *Capital Losses,* 15.

34. Constance McLaughlin Green, *Washington: A History of the Capital, 1800–1950* (Princeton, NJ: Princeton University Press, 1962), 82–84. On bankruptcy and honor, see Bruce A. Mann, *Republic of Debtors: Bankruptcy in the Age of American Independence* (Cambridge, MA: Harvard University Press, 2003); David A. Skeel Jr., *Debt's Dominion: A History of Bankruptcy Law in America* (Princeton, NJ: Princeton University Press, 2003); and Billy Smith, *Down and Out in Early America* (University Park, PA: Penn State Press, 2004).

35. The 1820 Georgetown census suggests the intriguing possibility that John moved there after Ann left him. During the period he remained in jail, the 1820 census contains notice of a "John Mattingley" under "Free Colored Persons" with a household of one male younger than fourteen and one male and one female between the ages of fourteen and twenty-six. Whether or not this free black family worked for John Mattingly, or simply shared a common name, is not known. It is possible that the black family was maintaining a house for John while he was in jail.

36. Mike Livingston, "Metropolitan Bank Keeps Up with Stately Neighbors," *Washington Business Journal,* October 8, 2004, http://www.bizjournals.com/washington/stories/2004/10/11/focus10.html (accessed August 10, 2010); "Fourth Census of the United States, 1820," NARA microfilm publication M33, Records of the Bureau of the Census, Record Group 29, National Archives and Records Administration, Washington, DC.

37. *National Intelligencer,* January 8, 1821, and January 18, 1822.

38. "A Bill, for the Relief of Insolvent Debtors within the District of Columbia" ([Washington City]: Duane and Sons, printers, 1802).

39. Green, *Washington: A History,* 88.

40. Ridout, "Peggy Stewart Tea Party Chapter," 459. Two of the cannons were placed at the students' entrance to Georgetown College in 1888, according to George P. Goff. A Georgetown student, C. Louis Palm, '89, composed the following poem about the cannon:

> Dark scowling bulks! O lumps of British ore!
> Moulded by hands that have returned to dust,
> Hallowed by two hundred years of rust!

Where's that fierce ring, that deafening crash of war
That long since echoed down St. Mary's shore?
You're mute, indeed, who once played slaves to Death,
Blasting the sons of men with hell's own breath.

Goff and poem quoted in James S. Easby-Smith, *Georgetown University in the District of Columbia, 1789–1907: Its Founders, Benefactors, Officers, Instructors and Alumni,* vol. 1 (Chicago: Lewis, 1907), 157.

41. Clark, "Mayors of the Corporation," 63–65.
42. *Metropolitan and Georgetown National Messenger,* June 6, 1822; Clark, "Mayors of the Corporation," 66–67. See also Green, *Washington: A History,* 88–89.
43. Green, *Washington: A History,* 89; Clark, "Mayors of the Corporation," 68.
44. Clark, "Mayors of the Corporation," 67–76.
45. "Presentment of the GAOL," Case Papers 1802–1863, June term 1818, rough bundle reports on the Washington, D.C., jail, Box 154, National Archives and Records Administration, Washington, DC.
46. Ibid., December term 1818, Judicials 243–301, Recognizances.
47. Ibid. These accounts, it should be noted, are in marked contrast to the description given by Anne Newport Royall during her visit to Washington in 1822, the same year John Mattingly would have been in the jail: "I found the prison of Washington under very different regulations from that of the poor house. Here I found health, cleanliness, and plenty of wholesome food; the prisoners cheerful and happy. I examined every cell that contained a criminal, which was twenty-four, and found neither despondency nor complaint. They were severally laughing, talking, and singing; and but for reality it would not appear that they were confined. The debtors' apartments are spacious and airy; and in no part of the prison did I witness any thing but the greatest tenderness and humanity toward those unfortunate beings. Much credit is due to the keeper, whoever he be, who thus does honor to himself, and to human nature." *Sketches of Life, History, and Manners in the United States by a Traveller* (1826), 143–144.
48. "John Mattingly, 10/22/1822," Record Group 21, Entry 26, Insolvent Case Papers, 1814–January 1842, National Archives and Records Administration, Washington, DC (special thanks to Robert Ellis of the National Archives for his assistance with these records); weather from Tessier, *Diary;* John Sessford, "Deaths in the City in 1822," *Records of the Columbia Historical Society* 11 (1908): 274–275.
49. The affidavit from Ruth and Catharine Carbery states that "during these six

years, she never left her bed for any considerable time, nor was out of her brother's house, but on two occasions: one when she was removed from his former to his present residence; the other, for the purpose of visiting an aged and favorite servant of the family, who was thought to be dying, and whose habitation was within ten yards of the door. That even in this short walk she needed and received assistance; and slight as that exercise was, it seemed greatly to affect her, as a copious puking of blood immediately followed it." Matthews, *Collection of Affidavits and Certificates,* 12.

Chapter 4. Thaumaturgus and Priest

1. A recent study of Johann Joseph Gassner is H. C. Erik Midelfort's excellent *Exorcism and Enlightenment: Johann Joseph Gassner and the Demons of Eighteenth-Century Germany* (New Haven, CT: Yale University Press, 2005). The story that opens this chapter is a synthesis of several cures and Gassner's techniques as described by Midelfort. Gassner's purported cures are also extensively discussed in F. A. Brodhaus, *Quintessenz aus den Wunderversuchen durch Michel und Hohenlohe* (Leipzig, 1822).

2. Midelfort, *Exorcism and Enlightenment,* 12–13, 67.

3. Ibid., 73.

4. On the Organic Edict, see Stephan Baron von Koskull, *Wunderglaube und Medizin, Die religiösen Heilungsversuche des Fürsten Alexander von Hohenlohe in Franken, 1821–1822* (Bamberg: Historischer Verein Bamberg Für die Pflege der Geschichte des ehemaligen Fürstbistums Bamberg, 22. Beiheft, 1988), 45–48.

5. Ibid., 49–54, 80.

6. Brodhaus, *Quintessenz aus den Wunderversuchen,* 7. Much of the biographical information here was drawn from Koskull, *Wunderglaube und Medizin,* who worked with an extensive collection of files of the Bavarian Department of Inner Affairs, now in the Bavarian main state archive in Munich. The file contains correspondence, official decrees, protocols of questionings, and medical reports concerning the attempts to cure that the Catholic priest Prince Alexander von Hohenlohe-Waldenburg-Schillingsfürst performed in 1821 and 1822 in Bamberg, Würzburg, and some other cities in Franken. Francis Nicholas Baur, in *A Short and Faithful Description of the Remarkable Occurrences and Benevolent Holy Conduct of His Serene Highness, Prince Alexander of Hohenlohe, Domicellar of Olmutz, Vicariat Counsellor of the See of Bamberg, and Knight of Malta, during his Residence of Twenty-four Days in the City of Würzburg in*

Twelve Confidential Letters, Translated from the German (Dublin: Richard Coyne, 1822), states that 1744 is the date of elevation of the family to the rank of Princes of the Holy Roman Empire by Charles VII.

7. Sebastian, *Fürst Alexander von Hohenlohe-Schillingsfürst*, 3–5; Karl Reichert, *Prinz Alexander von Hohenlohe: Ein "Wunderdoktor" zu Beginn des 19. Jahrhunderts. Ein Beitrag zur Medizingeschichte Frankens* (Dissertation, Julius-Maximilian-Universität, Würzburg, 1955), 2.

8. This biographical information is drawn from Burns, *American Phase.*

9. Georg Michael Pachtler, *Biographische Notizen über Seine Durchlaucht den hochseligen Prinzen Alexander zu Hohenlohe-Waldenburg-Schillingfürst, Bischof von Sardica* (Augsburg, 1850); Sebastian, *Alexander von Hohenlohe-Schillingsfürst*, 6–7.

10. Sebastian, *Alexander von Hohenlohe-Schillingsfürst*, 10.

11. Ibid., 9. The quotation is, "Quanto alla capacità, con molto mediocre talento egli ha fatto il corso de' studii con molta irregolarità ed infinite interruzzioni, e non essendovi giunta nessuna applicazione, la riuscita è stata poco più di nulla" (thanks to Rita Carter for her assistance with the translation from Italian), quoted in Koskull, *Wunderglaube und Medizin*, 7.

12. Sebastian, *Alexander von Hohenlohe-Schillingsfürst*, 11.

13. Bastgen, *Der Heilige Stuhl*, 7–8.

14. Ibid., 11–13, my translation.

15. Sebastian, *Alexander von Hohenlohe-Schillingsfürst*, 16–17.

16. Ibid., 19.

17. Ibid., 18–19.

18. On Severoli's allegation, see Bastgen, *Der Heilige Stuhl*, 24–25; Sebastian, *Alexander von Hohenlohe-Schillingsfürst*, 20–22; Burns, *American Phase*, 7.

19. Alexander von Hohenlohe-Schillingsfürst, *Abgedrungene Vertheidigung des Fürsten Alexander von Hohenlohe . . . gegen einen Aufsatz in dem Weimarer Oppositionsblatte vom Jahre 1819*, no. 73 (1819); Koskull, *Wunderglaube und Medizin*, 7.

20. Koskull, *Wunderglaube und Medizin*, 8, my translation.

21. Sebastian, *Alexander von Hohenlohe-Schillingsfürst*, 47; Thurston, "The Healing Hand," 323–333, 28.

22. Bastgen, *Der Heilige Stuhl*, 29–30.

23. Baur, *A Short and Faithful Description*, 5, 13; Bastgen, *Der Heilige Stuhl*, 31; Koskull, *Wunderglaube und Medizin*, 9.

24. Fischer, *Die merkwürdige Heilungsgeschichte*, 63–66, my translation.

25. Ludwig quoted in Baur, *A Short and Faithful Description*, 13–14; Sebastian,

Alexander von Hohenlohe-Schillingsfürst, 47–49; Fischer, *Die merkwürdige Heilungsgeschichte,* 22, my translation.

26. Sebastian, *Alexander von Hohenlohe-Schillingsfürst,* 48; Brodhaus, *Quintessenz aus den Wunderversuchen,* 96.

27. Koskull, *Wunderglaube und Medizin,* 9, 54, my translation.

28. Ibid., 26; Reichert, *Prinz Alexander von Hohenlohe,* 28, my translation.

29. Bastgen, *Der Heilige Stuhl,* 36, my translation.

30. Quoted in Koskull, *Wunderglaube und Medizin,* 30; Reichert, *Prinz Alexander von Hohenlohe,* 25, my translations.

31. C. G. Scharold, *Briefe aus Würzburg über die Wunderbaren Heilungen des Herrn Fürsten Alexander von Hohenlohe* (Würzburg, 1821), 4–5, my translation.

32. Ibid., 6–7, my translation; the detail about the prince's sweating is emphasized in Brodhaus, *Quintessenz aus den Wunderversuchen,* 143–144.

33. Koskull, *Wunderglaube und Medizin,* 26; Scharold, *Briefe aus Würzburg,* 13, 38–39.

34. Scharold, *Briefe aus Würzburg,* 51–52, my translation.

35. On the canonization process, see Jacalyn Duffin, *Medical Miracles: Doctors, Saints, and Healing in the Modern World* (London: Oxford University Press, 2009), esp. chapter 1.

36. Scharold, *Briefe aus Würzburg,* 52–53.

37. Bastgen, *Der Heilige Stuhl,* 38–39.

38. Ibid., 47–48.

39. Quoted in Brodhaus, *Quintessenz aus den Wunderversuchen,* 303–305, my translation; Reichert, *Prinz Alexander von Hohenlohe,* 31; *Neckar Zeitung,* September 16, 1821, quoted in Brodhaus, *Quintessenz aus den Wunderversuchen,* 305, my translation; Cassiodor Franz Joseph Zenger, *Vertrautes Gespräch über die vom Fürsten Alex. v. Hohenlohe gewirkten Heilungen* (Sulzbach, 1823), 26.

40. Koskull, *Wunderglaube und Medizin,* 31–35, my translations.

41. Ibid., 10.

42. Ibid.; Brodhaus, *Quintessenz aus den Wunderversuchen,* 201–212, 248–250.

43. Burns, *American Phase,* 13; Koskull, *Wunderglaube und Medizin,* 11.

44. Burns, *American Phase,* 14; Sebastian, *Alexander von Hohenlohe-Schillingsfürst,* 80–81; Lahner, *"Der Wunderdoktor,"* 11, states that Martin Michel developed the idea of setting aside a day and time to pray for people too sick to come to his village. Prince Hohenlohe expanded this idea of sending letters around the world.

45. Burns, *American Phase,* 14.

46. Friedrich Brenner, *Noch andere Ansichten von den Heilungen des Fürsten Alex-*

ander von Hohenlohe (1821), quoted in Reichert, *Prinz Alexander von Hohenlohe,* 58–59.

47. Quoted in Reichert, *Prinz Alexander von Hohenlohe,* 59–60.

48. Sebastian, *Alexander von Hohenlohe-Schillingsfürst,* 139. Sebastian's source
appears to be Feuerbach, L. Anselm Ritter von Feuerbach Biographic Estate,
Collected Papers Leipzig in 1853, vol. II, 166 ff. Duke L is identified as Duke
von Rechteren-Limpourg.

49. "Prince Hohenlohe's Miraculous Cures," in *The Book of Days: A Miscellany
of Popular Antiquities,* ed. R. Chambers (1869), http://www.thebookofdays
.com/months/march/16.htm (accessed August 13, 2010).

50. Ibid.

51. John Badeley, *Authentic Narrative of the Extraordinary Cure Performed by
Prince Alexandre Hohenlohe on Miss Barbara O'Connor, a Nun, in the Convent
of New Hall, near Chelmsford; with a Full Refutation of the Numerous False
Reports and Misrepresentations,* 2nd ed. (London, 1823), 15 (description of
the ailment).

52. James Doyle, O.S.A., *An Account of a Miracle Wrought by Prince de Hohenlohe
(Priest of the Catholic Church) the 10th of June, 1823 on Miss Maria Lalor, of
Rosskilton, Who Had Been Dumb for Six Years and Five Months* (Manchester,
1823). For a comprehensive discussion of this and other Irish cures, see Lau-
rence M. Geary, "Prince Hohenlohe, Signor Pastorini and Miraculous Healing
in Early Nineteenth-Century Ireland," in *Medicine, Disease and the State in
Ireland, 1650–1940,* ed. Greta Jones and Elizabeth Malcolm (Cork, Ireland:
Cork University Press, 1999), 40–58.

53. Geary, "Prince Hohenlohe, Signor Pastorini and Miraculous Healing," 43–45.

54. Ibid., 53; *Warder,* July 5, 1823; on O'Connell, see ibid., 48–49.

55. Quoted in Geary, "Prince Hohenlohe, Signor Pastorini and Miraculous Healing," 50.

56. "Lord Norbery and the Irish Miracle," *Miscellaneous Cabinet,* November 22,
1823, 1, 20, 160.

57. Koskull, *Wunderglaube und Medizin,* 74.

Chapter 5. A Capital Miracle

1. This story of the Livingston haunting, which various sources date as occurring
between 1789 and 1797, is a synthesis of the tale from several sources, including
the following: James E. Harding, "United States Department of the Interior
Historic Conservation and Recreation Service, National Register of Historic

Places Inventory, Nomination Form: Smithfield, Middleway, Wizard Clip,"
http://www.wvculture.org/shpo/nr/pdf/jefferson/80004025.pdf; "Ghosts of
the Prairie: The Livingston Wizard," http://www.prairieghosts.com/wizard
.html; W. S. Laidley, "'Wizzard Clip' (Wizard Clip)," *West Virginia Historical
Magazine Quarterly*, January 1904, http://www.wvculture.org/History/notewv/
wizardclip1.html (all accessed August 15, 2010); John Gilmary Shea, *Life and
Times of the Most Rev. John Carroll, Bishop and First Archbishop of Baltimore
Embracing the History of the Catholic Church in the United States, 1763–1815*
(New York: John G. Shea, 1888), 288–290. For a full account, see Joseph Maria
Finotti, *The Mystery of the Wizard Clip* (Baltimore, MD: Kelly, Piet, 1879).
The story is also retold in *A Diary of Br. Joseph Mobberly*, vol. IV, Memo-
randum, 1824, Jesuit Plantation Project: Maryland's Jesuit Plantations, 1650–
1838, 71–94, http://www8.georgetown.edu/departments/americanstudies/
jpp/diary4.html (accessed August 15, 2010). The detail about the sour milk and
the Methodist minister is from Rev. Peter Henry Lemcke, O.S.B., *Life and
Work of Prince Demetrius Augustine Gallitzin*, trans. Rev. Joseph C. Plumpe
(New York: Longmans, Green, 1940), 124–126. For a new treatment of this
story and the role of Gallitzin, see John R. Dichtl, *Frontiers of Faith: Bringing Catholicism to the West in the Early Republic* (Lexington: University Press
of Kentucky, 2008), 114–116; Sarah M. Brownson, *Life of Demetrius Augustine Gallitzin, Prince and Priest* (1873), 100–108; and Daniel Sargent, *Mitri,
or the Story of Prince Demetrius Augustine Gallitzin, 1770–1840* (New York:
Longmans, Green, 1945), 113–116. Gallitzin's compliment to Cahill ("man of
powerful nerve") is quoted in Thomas W. Spalding, *The Premier See: A History of the Archdiocese of Baltimore, 1789–1994* (Baltimore, MD: Johns Hopkins
University Press, 1989), 35.

2. Brian Alderson, "The Spoken and the Read: German Popular Stories and
English Popular Diction," in *The Reception of Grimm's Fairy Tales: Responses,
Reactions, Revisions*, ed. Donald Haase (Detroit: Wayne State University Press,
1993), 63–65.

3. "Miracles," *City Gazette and Commercial Daily Advertiser*, Charleston, SC,
November 1, 1821; "Prince Hohenlohe," *United States Catholic Miscellany* 1, no.
19 (October 9, 1822), 146; "Latest from England," *Alexandria* (VA) *Herald*, May
5, 1823; "The Dublin Journal of the 5th," *Ithaca* (NY) *Journal*, November 5,
1823; "Prince Hohenlohe," *United States Catholic Miscellany* 4, no. 1 (January
5, 1824), 11; untitled article, *Boston Medical Intelligencer* 1, no. 34 (January 6,
1824), 134; "Edinburgh Review," *Rhode-Island American*, Providence, Feb-

ruary 10, 1824; and "Prince Hohenlohe," *City Gazette and Commercial Daily Advertiser,* Charleston, SC, February 23, 1824.

4. The dates of the *London Times* articles: September 13, 1821; April 20, 1822; March 13, August 6, August 23, August 29 ("regarding the pretended miracles"), September 6, September 9, November 25, and December 2, 1823. A satire of the prince's miracles was also published January 21, 1825. The *Monthly Repository of Theology and General Literature,* January to December 1822, vol. 17, ed. George Smallfield, 400–403. See "Lord Norbery and the Irish Miracle," *Miscellaneous Cabinet,* November 22, 1823, 1, 20, 160; "Valentine," *New Monthly Magazine and Literary Journal,* American ed., 1824, 8, 46, 327, a poem that states, "And we have seen Prince Hohenlohe has fail'd / In his impostures and his Irish trade."

5. Letter to Mrs. Dickenson, St. Thomas Manor, Portobacco, Charles County, MD, October 20, 1822, archives of the Georgetown Visitation Monastery.

6. Information about the Carbery family can be found in Clark, "Mayors of the Corporation," 61–98.

7. For an excellent discussion of lay trusteeism, see Randall M. Miller, "A Church in Cultural Captivity: Some Speculations on Catholic Identity in the Old South," in *Catholics in the Old South: Essays on Church and Culture,* ed. Randall M. Miller and Jon L. Wakelyn (Macon, GA: Mercer University Press, 1983), 20–29.

8. William W. Warner, *At Peace with All Their Neighbors: Catholics and Catholicism in the Nation's Capital, 1787–1860* (Washington, DC: Georgetown University Press, 1994), esp. chapter 8.

9. Grassi quoted in ibid., 147; Spalding, *The Premier See,* 17–18.

10. Spalding, *The Premier See,* 17–20.

11. Quoted in ibid., 54; on Matthews, see ibid., 60–62; Christopher J. Kauffman, *Tradition and Transformation in Catholic Culture: The Priests of St. Sulpice in the United States from 1791 to the Present* (New York: Macmillan, 1988), and quoted in Spalding, *The Premier See,* 63.

12. On Neale, see Spalding, *The Premier See,* 75–77; Maréchal quoted at 80.

13. On the trustee battle, see ibid., 81–82; "Letter to Thomas Jefferson" at 82.

14. The Paine story is repeated in J. Wilfred Parsons, "Rev. Anthony Kohlmann, S.J. (1771–1824)," *Catholic Historical Review* 4 (April 1918): 38–51.

15. Robert Emmett Curran, *The Bicentennial History of Georgetown University: From Academy to University, 1789–1889,* vol. I (Washington, DC: Georgetown University Press, 1993), 85.

16. Thomas Murphy, S.J., *Jesuit Slaveholding in Maryland, 1717–1838* (New York:

Routledge, 2001), 165. Murphy makes the point that Kohlmann feared a "drift too far toward American republicanism and individualism" (167).

17. Kohlmann and Archbishop Maréchal had another well-documented tiff, the nine-year-long pension, or stipend, controversy that flared in 1820, see Spalding, *The Premier See,* 84–85; on Maréchal's trip to Rome, see Spalding, *The Premier See,* 88. Discussion of the controversies also appears in Curran, *Bicentennial History,* 84–99. On the property challenge and the complaint of the trustees, see Spalding, *The Premier See,* 90, 92.

18. Letter from Stephen Dubuisson to Ambrose Maréchal, August 30, 1821, AAB, 16, B1.

19. Letter from Stephen Dubuisson to Prince Hohenlohe, January 2, 1824 (draft), Georgetown University Library, Special Collections Division, Washington, DC, MPA, 19, D1, quoted in Curran, "'The Finger of God,'" 43; letter from John Beschter to "Rev. & Dr Father in Christ" [Dubuisson], Baltimore, February 6, 1824, MPA, 13, 16; letter from Stephen Dubuisson to William Beschter, February 10, 1824, MPA, 13, 16.

20. Letter from Ambrose Maréchal to Stephen Dubuisson, Baltimore, February 13, 1824, AAB, 16, B5. See also letter from Maréchal to Dubuisson, Baltimore, February 13, 1824, MPA, 13, 16.

21. Letter from Maréchal to William Matthews, March 12, 1824, AAB, quoted in Burns, *American Phase,* 26–27, and partially quoted in Curran, "'Finger of God,'" 45. On Maréchal's fear, see Spalding, *The Premier See,* 99.

22. Letter from William Matthews to Archbishop Maréchal, March 19, 1824, AAB, quoted in Burns, *American Phase,* 21. The four petitioners are named in a letter from Stephen Dubuisson to William Beschter, February 10, 1824, MPA, 13, 16. Boone and Wimsatt are mentioned in a letter from Foster on behalf of Prince Hohenlohe dated May 7, 1824, MPA, 60, 6. Anthony Kohlmann, affidavit, March 20, 1824, in Matthews, *Collection of Affidavits and Certificates.* On Tessier's participation and Matthews' report of March 19, 1824, to Archbishop Maréchal, see Burns, *American Phase,* 22.

23. Details about the towel and laudanum are found in Clark, "Mayors of the Corporation," 81–82; the letter from Prince Hohenlohe is quoted in Burns, *American Phase,* 23.

24. Letter from Stephen Dubuisson to Francis Dzierozynski, March 10, 1824, MPA, quoted in Burns, *American Phase,* 24, who mistakes the name as "James Druiserynsky"; letter from William Matthews to Ambrose Maréchal, March 10, 1824, AAB, 19, B15, quoted in Burns, *American Phase,* 24–26, and in Curran,

"'Finger of God,'" 45; draft of letter from Dubuisson to Prince Hohenlohe, March 11, 1824, MPA, 13, 16; Tessier, *Diary,* March 10, 1824.

25. Letter from Ambrose Maréchal to William Matthews, March 12, 1824, quoted in Burns, *American Phase,* 26–27, and partially quoted in Curran, "'Finger of God,'" 45.

26. Letter from Thomas Carbery to Ambrose Maréchal, Washington, March 13, 1824, AAB, 14, B1, quoted in Curran, "'Finger of God,'" 45; letter from Kohlmann to ?, Georgetown, March 12, 1824, MPA, 206, P23, quoted in Curran, "'Finger of God,'" 46n; letter from Kohlmann to Lewis Wilcocks, White Marsh, March 16, 1824, published in the *Baltimore Federal Gazette,* March 27, 1824, and republished in the *National Intelligencer,* April 3, 1824; letter from Francis Dzierozynski to Father Epinette, March 13, 1824, MPA 93, 5. See also letter from Father John Odin to M. Challeton, 1824, in *Annales de l'association de la propagation de la foi,* II, 367, quoted in Burns, *American Phase,* 28.

27. The Navy Yard story can be found in a letter from William Matthews to Ambrose Maréchal, Washington, March 19, 1824, AAB, 19, B16, quoted in Curran, "'Finger of God,'" 46n; *National Gazette and Literary Register,* March 20, 1824, Philadelphia.

28. Letter from Matthews to Maréchal, Washington, March 19, 1824, AAB, 19, B16, also quoted in Burns, *American Phase,* 33; letter from Ambrose Maréchal to Stephen Dubuisson, Baltimore, March 31, 1824, MPA, 13, 16.

29. "A Miracle," *Salem* (MA) *Gazette,* March 19, 1924.

30. The eighteen newspaper articles reviewed from 1824 are as follows: "A Miracle," *Salem* (MA) *Gazette,* March 19; "Miracles," *Portsmouth* (NH) *Journal of Literature and Politics,* March 20; untitled, *Baltimore* (MD) *Patriot,* March 22; untitled, *Boston Commercial Gazette,* March 22; "New York, March 10, Extraordinary Cure," *Rhode-Island American,* March 23, Providence; "Prince Hohenlohe in America," *Richmond* (VA) *Enquirer,* March 23; "The Miracle," *Salem* (MA) *Gazette,* March 23; "Died," *City Gazetteer and Commercial Advertiser,* March 24, Charleston, SC; untitled, *New London* (CT) *Gazette and General Advertiser,* March 24; "Prince Hohenlohe's Miracle in Washington," *Richmond* (VA) *Enquirer,* March 26; untitled, *Haverhill* (MA) *Gazette & Patriot,* March 27; "The Miracle," *Essex Register,* March 29, Salem, MA; "The Days of St. Patrick and the Snakes Returned," *Watch-Tower,* March 29, Cooperstown, NY; "The Age of Miracles," *North Star,* March 30, Danville, VT; untitled, *Rhode-Island American,* March 30, Providence; "Prince Hohenlohe," *Salem* (MA) *Gazette,* March 30; "The Miracle," *New London* (CT) *Gazette & General Advertiser,* March 31; untitled, *Providence* (RI) *Gazette,* March 21.

31. "Humbug," *Haverhill* (MA) *Gazette & Patriot,* May 8, 1824; "From the Evening Post," *Saratoga Sentinel,* June 8, 1824, Saratoga Springs, NY.

32. Quotation from *Mount Zion Missionary* and Guilday's observation can be found in Peter Guilday, *The Life and Times of John England,* vol. II (New York: Arno Press, 1969), 426.

33. "The Hohenlohe Miracle," *Boston Commercial Gazette,* June 24, 1824. On the idea of "a limited age of miracles," see Robert Bruce Mullin, *Miracles and the Modern Imagination* (New Haven, CT: Yale University Press, 1996), esp. chapters 1 and 2. Although many Protestant leaders such as the educated Episcopalian William Hawley dismissed miracles as a modern phenomenon, the Protestant masses began a turning toward the supernatural that would flower in the second half of the nineteenth century. According to the website of St. John's Church (http://www.stjohns-dc.org/article.php?id=48), the church's bell, cast in Boston by Paul Revere's son, Joseph, was installed in the church on November 30, 1822. In a strange historical coincidence, the first ringing of the bell was on the day Ann's husband, John Mattingly, died. Adherents to Protestantism were likely practicing forms of religious folk magic, as the story of Joseph Smith, the founder of Mormonism attests. Just one year before Ann Mattingly's miraculous cure, Smith claimed to have been visited by the Angel Moroni, who revealed the location of the golden plates of Cumorah. When measuring the Protestant response to the Mattingly miracle of 1824, it is instructive to remember that this splintering off of a major Protestant sect after a supernatural event began the year before, in 1823.

34. Chrysostom, "Miraculous Cures," *Washington Theological Repertory,* April 1, 1824, 327.

35. See *Reformer,* May 1, 1824, 5, 53, 105, and July 1, 1824, 5, 55, 165; and "An Examination of a Protestant's Objections," *Orthodox Journal,* May 1824, MPA, 14, 1.

36. "An Examination of a Protestant's Objections." The retort from the Preston Catholic Defense Society was immediate and seething: "The writer signs himself '*A Protestant,*' which may mean anything or nothing, for he may be a deist, an atheist, a ranter, a jumper, a muggletonian, or a huggletonian, a jew, a turk, or an infidel, provided he protests against the doctrines of the church of Rome." The British Catholic writer extols Kohlmann as an accomplished scholar and priest and takes on the question, Why America? But the underlying theme of his answer is also the polarity, skepticism *versus* belief: "And what greater authority do we want to convince the rational mind of the actual occurrence of the miracle? Here is the sister of the first civil magistrate of the first city

of a people enjoying perfect freedom, both civil and religious, miraculously cured of an inveterate disease; she is seen and congratulated by thousands of persons, all in possession of the liberty of the press, and therefore capable of detecting fraud, while fraud is defied to be proved; and what more can be required to carry conviction to the unprejudiced man?" From the viewpoint of a British writer, Washington was an important setting, and the large amount of press coverage of the miracle enhanced its truth. The writer from the Catholic Defense Society insists that the miracles are signs that the Catholic Church is the True Church. The pamphlet concludes: "here we have the ministers of the Catholic church, who alone possess an uninterrupted succession from the apostles, invoking the sacred name of Jesus, in behalf of the sick, and the sick recover; these ministers preach the world every where, and in France, Germany, England, Ireland, and America, the *word* they preach is *confirmed,* with *signs* that follow, the *Lord working* withal. These signs are attested by indubitable witnesses; they are disputed by incredulity, but not disproved." The sectarian battles over the "ownership" of God's special grace are at the base—a question of faith and belief versus skepticism over supernatural signs.

37. "Prince Hohenlohe—The Miracle-Monger," *Salem* (MA) *Gazette,* July 21, 1829; "Prince Hohenlohe has ceased to work miracles . . . ," *Independent Inquirer,* April 19, 1834, Brattleboro, VT; *Southern Patriot,* May 1, 1834, Charleston, SC; *Macon* (GA) *Weekly Telegraph–Georgia Telegraph,* May 5, 1834; *Haverhill* (MA) *Gazette–Essex Gazette,* May 24, 1834; *Ladies' Companion, a Monthly Magazine* (July 1834), 1, 3, 116, and "Rev. Prince Alexander of Hohenlohe," *Baltimore Literary and Religious Magazine* (March 1835), 1, 3, 83. On the Ursuline Convent attack, see Nancy Lusignan Schultz, *Fire and Roses: The Burning of the Charlestown Convent, 1834* (New York: Free Press, 2000).

38. Curran, "'The Finger of God,'" 48. Curran states that Dubuisson suspected Levins, which is probably the case. He does not, however, pursue the trail of Rev. Hawley, also mentioned. See notes on the Refutation Pamphlet, MPA, 19, D1, unsigned, but in the handwriting of Stephen Dubuisson. Dubuisson writes, "The fact is Mr. Hawley, a few days before it appeared, boasted of being on the point of refuting the miraculous fabrick." Draft of letter to Ambrose Maréchal, MPA, 14, 1.

39. Guilday, *The Life and Times of John England,* 427–431. For the full series of Bishop John England's response to Rev. William Hawley, see Ignatius Aloysius Reynolds, "Letters of Various Misrepresentations of the Catholic Religion. Addressed to the Rev. William Hawley," in *The Works of the Right Rev. John England, Bishop of Charleston,* vol. II, 213–277. Friend of Truth, *The*

Washington Miracle Refuted: Or, a Review of the Rev. Mr. Matthew's Pamphlet (Georgetown, DC, 1824), 1.

40. Friend of Truth, *Miracle Refuted,* 37.

41. Ibid., 7, 9.

42. Ibid., 25; "seraphic Kohlman," 5; "modern Thaumaturgus," 6.

43. Ibid., 23.

44. Ibid., 36–37, 41.

45. Quoted in Burns, *American Phase,* 33n.

46. Letter from Anthony Kohlmann to Lewis Wilcocks, March 16, 1824, in *Baltimore Federal Gazette,* March 27, 1824.

47. "To the Editors: A Card," *National Intelligencer,* March 30, 1824.

48. Letter from William Matthews to Ambrose Maréchal, March 31, 1824, AAB, 29, B18, quoted in Burns, *American Phase,* 29–30, and Curran, "'Finger of God,'" 46.

49. Letter of Democritus, *National Intelligencer,* April 1, 1824.

50. Ibid.

51. Ibid.

52. Quoted in Curran, "'Finger of God,'" 48.

53. "A Catholic Layman," *National Intelligencer,* April 5, 1824.

54. Letter of Democritus.

55. Letter from Thomas C. Levins to Roger Baxter, April 7, 1824, MPA, 60, 5.

56. Ibid.

57. Letter from Thomas C. Levins to Joseph Carbery, April 15, 1824, MPA, 60, 5.

58. Letters from William Beschter to Stephen Dubuisson, Baltimore, March 24 and July 14, 1824, MPA, 14, 1. A similar sentiment is expressed in Beschter's letter to Dubuisson on July 10, 1824, MPA, 14, 1.

59. Letter from Stephen Dubuisson to Ambrose Maréchal, Baltimore, July 10, 1824, MPA, 19, D1.

60. Letter from Anthony Kohlmann to Peter Kenney, New York, 23 May, 1824, MPA, 60, 6. In the same letter, Kohlmann alludes to the return of William Hogan from Europe, who caused a schism in Philadelphia.

61. *Diary of Brother Mobberly,* vol. IV, 1–3.

62. Ibid., December 23, 1824; letter of dismissal from Aloysius Fortis to Thomas Levins, October 1824, MPA, 60, 4.

63. *Diary of Brother Mobberly,* 23; letter from Peter Chotard to Stephen Dubuisson, Baltimore, November 1, 1824, MPA, 14, 1.

64. Letter from Archbishop Maréchal to Archbishop Plessis, Georgetown, May 16, 1824, in "Maréchal: Correspondence," 455–459.

65. Jacalyn Duffin, *Medical Miracles: Doctors, Saints and Healing in the Modern World* (Oxford: Oxford University Press, 2009), chapter 5; letter from Stephen Dubuisson to John England, March 11, 1824, MPA, 14, 1.

66. Matthews, *Collection of Affidavits and Certificates,* 7; letter from Thomas Carbery to John England, Washington City, April 8, 1826, MPA, 13, 6.

67. Matthews, *Collection of Affidavits and Certificates,* 13. I am grateful to Dr. Maura McGrane for consulting with me on the symptoms of Ann Mattingly's illness.

68. Ibid., 16, 19, 20. On "victim souls," see Paula Kane, "'She Offered Herself Up': The Victim Soul and Victim Spirituality in Catholicism," *Church History* 71, no. 1 (March 2002).

69. Matthews, *Collection of Affidavits and Certificates,* 41.

70. England, *Works,* vol. III, 393.

71. Ibid., 394.

72. Ibid., 397.

73. Ibid., 397, 404; Jenny Franchot, *Roads to Rome: The Antebellum Protestant Encounter with Catholicism* (Berkeley: University of California Press, 2004), 23–25.

74. England, *Works,* vol. III, 400, 395.

75. Letter from Stephen Dubuisson to Bishop England, fragment, I-II, August 1828, MPA, 13, 16. He did send a letter in Latin to Benedict Fenwick from the College of Rome where he was stationed about Mrs. Mattingly's *odor Christie,* September 6, 1828, MPA, 61, 24.

76. England, *Works,* vol. III, 395, 398; Ray Allen Billington, *The Protestant Crusade, 1800–1860: A Study of the Origins of American Nativism* (New York: Macmillan, 1938).

Chapter 6. Aftermath

1. Donald B. Webster Jr., "The beauty and chivalry of the United States assembled . . . ," *American Heritage Magazine* 17, no. 1 (December 1965), AmericanHeritage.com, http://www.americanheritage.com/articles/magazine/ah/1965/1/1965_1_50.shtml (accessed August 17, 2010). Both Webster and Lincoln P. Paine, *Warships of the World to 1900* (New York: Houghton Mifflin, 2000), 136, assert that the hull was made of iron.

2. Webster, "beauty and chivalry."

3. Ibid.

4. *National Intelligencer,* March 4, 1844.

5. From material in private family collection. Virgil Maxcy Mattingly, called "Joseph Mattingley" in cemetery records, was born in Washington, D.C., and is buried at Glenwood Cemetery. See Wesley E. Pippenger, *District of Columbia Interments (Index to Deaths), January 1, 1855 to July 31, 1874* (Westminster, MD: Willow Bend, 1999), 235.

6. Ann Taves, *The Household of Faith: Roman Catholic Devotions in Mid-Nineteenth-Century America* (Notre Dame, IN: University of Notre Dame Press, 1986), 103, and Marie Pagliarini, "And the Word Was Made Flesh": Divining the Female Body in Nineteenth-Century American and Catholic Culture," *Religion and American Culture* 17, no. 2 (summer 2007): 213–245, 218.

7. The prayer is quoted in Curran, "'Finger of God,'" 41–61, 44n. One important distinction between the European and American cures by Hohenlohe involved the role that the Eucharist played in the cures. In Europe, the cure was most often accomplished at the moment the Host was elevated during consecration. In the American cures, the vital moment was the actual swallowing of the Host, as though Jesus had to be physically encountered for the cure to be effected. Curran also makes the point about the physical encounter (57).

8. Barbara Welter, "The Cult of True Womanhood: 1820–1860," *American Quarterly* 18, no. 2, part I (summer 1966): 151–174; Paula Kane, James Kenneally, and Karen Kenneally, eds., *Gender Identities in American Catholicism* (Maryknoll, NY: Orbis, 2001), xix–1.

9. England, *Works,* vol. III, 394.

10. Pagliarini, "And the Word Was Made Flesh," 224; Friend of Truth, *Miracle Refuted,* 28; Eberebron the Pilgrim, *National Journal,* October 28, 1824, quoted in *Diary of Brother Mobberly,* November 19, 1824; *Sermons of Father J. P. Clorivière,* April 19, 1824, Book 8, 28, Georgetown Visitation Archives, and excerpted in Pagliarini, "And the Word Was Made Flesh," 233.

11. Pagliarini, "And the Word Was Made Flesh," 214; for Fanny Burney's account, see "Old Tyme Mastectomy," from *Eyewitness to History,* ed. John Carey, http://wesclark.com/jw/mastectomy.html (accessed May 5, 2010); for a theoretical discussion of Burney, see Julia L. Epstein, "Writing the Unspeakable: Fanny Burney's Mastectomy and the Fictive Body," *Representations* 16 (Autumn 1986): 131–166.

12. Susan Sontag, *Illness as Metaphor and AIDS and Its Metaphors* (New York: Picador, 2001), 9–10.

13. Ibid., 21–23.

14. Guy quoted in Samuel J. Kowal, "Emotions as a Cause of Cancer: 18th and

19th Century Contributions," *Psychoanalytic Review* 24, no. 3 (July 1955): 217–227, 219; William Buchan, "Of a Scirrhus and Cancer," in *Domestic Medicine* (1785), http://americanrevolution.org/medicine/med45.html (accessed August 18, 2010); for an excellent synopsis of the shifting historical perceptions of breast cancer, see James S. Olson, *Bathsheba's Breast: Women, Cancer & History* (Baltimore, MD: Johns Hopkins University Press, 2002).

15. Buchan, "Of a Scirrhus and Cancer," quoted in Robert N. Aronowitz, *Unnatural History: Breast Cancer and American Society* (Cambridge: Cambridge University Press, 2007), 24.

16. See *discipline* and *mortification* in Donald Attwater, ed., *A Catholic Dictionary*, 3rd ed. (Rockford, IL: Tan, 1958), 150, 333.

17. The origin of this discussion of the body and society is strongly influenced by Michelle Brandwein's discussion of Daniel Defoe's *A Journal of the Plague Year*, in which she notes that "the body depends on society for its survival, yet by virtue of its foreignness from it must struggle against it. The body is society's precursor: the body with its needs and desires existed before language, intellectual activity, culture, and societal institutions and laws. The body was a whole before it was a part (of society). Bodily illness is thus a potential lever for exposing a society's insecurity." Michelle Brandwein, "Formation, Process, and Transition in *A Journal of the Plague Year*," in *Daniel Defoe's* A Journal of the Plague Year, ed. Paula R. Backscheider (New York: W. W. Norton, 1992), 340.

18. John England, *Letters to the Hon. John Forsyth on the Subject of Domestic Slavery* (Baltimore, 1844); Miller, "A Church in Cultural Captivity," 7.

19. R. Emmett Curran, "'Splendid Poverty': Jesuit Slaveholding in Maryland, 1805–1838," in *Catholics in the Old South*, 126n, 126.

20. Ibid., 127. See also Loretta M. Butler and Jacqueline E. Wilson, *O Write My Name: African-American Catholics in the Archdiocese of Washington, 1634–1990*, 2nd ed. (Washington, DC: Archdiocese of Washington, 2000), 9.

21. Curran, "'Splendid Poverty,'" 128–129.

22. Ibid., 134–135 ("since the great stir," 134).

23. Ibid.; letter from Anthony Kohlmann to Peter Kenney, New York, May 1824, MPA, 60, 6.

24. Letter from Aloysius Fortis to Dzierozynski, March 25, 1824, MPA, 500, 39b, quoted in Curran, "'Splendid Poverty,'" 135; Thomas Hughes, S.J., *The History of the Society of Jesus in North America: Colonial and Federal: Documents*, 2 vols. (London, 1908), vol. 1., 379–380, quoted in Curran, "'Splendid Poverty,'" 135n, 136.

25. *Diary of Brother Mobberly,* vol. 1., 143; Curran, "'Splendid Poverty,'" 131; Richard R. Duncan, "Catholics and the Church in the Antebellum Upper South," in *Catholics in the Old South,* 89. See also Butler and Wilson, *Write My Name,* 10.

26. Curran, "'Splendid Poverty,'" 131–132.

27. Warner, *At Peace,* 106.

28. John Gilmary Shea, *Memorial of the First Centenary of Georgetown College, D.C. comprising a History of Georgetown University* (New York: P. F. Collier, 1891), 65. See also James S. Easby-Smith, *Georgetown University in the District of Columbia, 1789–1907: Its Founders, Benefactors, Officers, Instructors and Alumni,* vol. 1 (New York and Chicago: Lewis, 1907), 59, and "Reminiscences of Dr. DeLoughery, A.B. 1826," *College Journal* 14, no. 5 (February 1886): 50–51, available in the Georgetown University Archives, Special Collections.

29. Dubuisson, "Mrs. Mattingly's Affair," MPA, 14, 1.

30. Ibid.; letter of dismissal from Aloysius Fortis to Thomas Levins, October 1824, MPA, 60, 4.

31. "Georgetown College Annual Commencement, Thursday, the 28th of July, 1825, at 3 O'Clock P.M.," program in Georgetown University Archives; Easby-Smith, *Georgetown University,* 60.

32. Easby-Smith, *Georgetown University,* 61. The students who performed included George Anderson, Thomas Walsh, Alexander Dimitry, Robert J. Brent, and Solomon Hillen. The student who read the Declaration of Independence was Theodore Jenkins, of Maryland.

33. Shea, *History of Georgetown University,* 71.

34. Ibid., 73–74.

35. Moore, "Epistle," 101.

36. Samuel Kercheval, *A History of the Valley of Virginia,* 2nd ed. (Woodstock, VA: John Gatewood, 1850); Alvin Edward Moore, *History of Hardy County of the Borderland* (Parsons, WV: McClain, 1963), 66–67.

37. John R. Wennersten, "A Capital Waterfront: Maritime Washington, D.C., 1790–1880," 1–40, 18–19, http://www.nmhf.org/pdf/capital_waterfront.pdf (accessed August 19, 2010).

38. Letter from Thomas Carbery to Rev. Dubuisson, May 16, 1828, MPA, 14, 1.

39. Letter from Ann Mattingly to Rev. Dubuisson, May 22, 1828, MPA, 14, 1.

40. Frank Graziano, in a recent book, *Wounds of Love: The Mystical Marriage of St. Rose of Lima* (New York: Oxford University Press, 2004), insists that although scholars such as Carolyn Walker Bynum have downplayed the eroticism of late medieval spiritual mysticism, it is highly erotic and "ludicrous" to deny

it: "One would have to dismiss or view in a very particular light the nuptial imagery of mystical marriage, including the semi-naked Bridegroom who offers and receives caresses, the brides who forfeit their virginity in Christ's heavenly bedchamber, and the burning love described by mystics who incorporate Christ's body. One would also have to ignore, neutralize, or apologize for the innumerable beatas, nuns, and female saints who report having kissed Christ on his mouth and body, who strip naked before the crucifix, who drink from Christ's wound as though it were a breast, who have lascivious visions of otherworldly seducers, and who have copulation ecstacies and masturbation fantasies with Christ as their subject" (10).

41. John R. Dichtl, *Frontiers of Faith: Bringing Catholicism to the West in the Early Republic* (Lexington: University Press of Kentucky, 2008), 116, 140–141.

42. *United States Federal Census,* Georgetown, Washington, DC, Roll 14, page 182. Baptismal records from St. Patrick's Church in the 1830s complicate the sorting out of John's marriage to Harriet, since two John Mattinglys appear in the records, married to two seemingly different Harriets—a Harriet Watts and a Harriet Doyle. The two John Mattinglys in Washington appear to have lived nearly parallel lives. On September 20, 1831, seven-month-old Charles was baptized, son of John Mattingly and Harriet Watts. This John Mattingly, a blacksmith, married Harriet Watts in Washington, June 14, 1827, just twelve days after the birth of Thomas Joseph Mattingly in Moorefield, western Virginia. The blacksmith John Mattingly signed his name on a land deed in 1828 with an X mark, which in my view rules him out as the Georgetown-educated son of Ann Mattingly. In another bizarre coincidence, this same land deed was examined and delivered to an official on September 23, 1839, the same year as family records indicate that John Baptist Carbery Mattingly died. Deed of Trust between Mr. & Mrs. John Mattingly & Mr. Matthew Delaney, WB no. 23, 1828 Old BX6, New 283, *D.C. Indentures of Apprenticeship,* 1801–1893, November 11, 1819. During my hunt for both John Mattinglys, father and son, I encountered many of their doppelgangers in the historical record, a challenge of working with a common name. On August 23, 1823, John, baby son of John Mattingly and Harriet Doyle, born on December 6, 1832, was baptized at St. Patrick's Church, with Louisa Mattingly as his sponsor. Both surviving children of John Baptist Carbery Mattingly and his wife Harriet, Thomas Joseph and Annie Elizabeth, named their daughters Harriet. St. Patrick's Baptismal Register, 1819–December 1836, 255, 301.

43. Letter from Ann Mattingly to Stephen Dubuisson, August 5, 1830, MPA, 62, 18.

44. "John Mattingly, 02/29/1832," Record Group 21, Entry 26, Insolvent Case Papers, 1814–January 1842, National Archives and Records Administration, Washington, DC.

45. Ibid.

46. St. Patrick's Baptismal Register, 302. The record states, "Aug. 23, 1833—John, son of John Mattingly and Harriet Doyle, his wife, born December 6, 1832. Sponsor: Louisa Mattingly"; "Deaths in Eighteen Hundred Thirty-Nine," *Records of the Columbia Historical Society,* vol. 11, 317. Thanks to Elizabeth Culhane and Paul Mattingly for help with obtaining this record.

47. England, *Works,* vol. I, 149.

48. *United States Catholic Miscellany,* June 8, 1825, reprinted in England, *Works,* vol. III, 476.

49. *Miraculous Cure of Sister Beatrix Meyers, a Nun of the Visitation in Georgetown* (Washington, DC, 1825), 4.

50. Letter from Mother Rose White to Archbishop Maréchal, June 21, 1826, AAB, quoted in Burns, *American Phase,* 54; letter from Mother Rose to Archbishop Maréchal, August 20, 1826, AAB, 69; letter from Sister Josephine Collins to Archbishop Maréchal, July 15, 1827, quoted in Burns, *American Phase,* 69.

51. *Narrative of Two Wonderful Cures Wrought in the Convent of the Visitation at Georgetown in the District of Columbia, in the Month of January, 1831* (Baltimore, 1831), 19; Burns, *American Phase,* 73–74.

52. Curran, "'Finger of God,'" 53n; Clorivière quoted in Pagliarini, "And the Word Was Made Flesh," 218.

53. Curran writes, "No one tracked the charts of the cured as persistently as did Dubuisson. He secured accounts of the miracles from the cured persons themselves, whenever possible. As late as 1862 he was writing from Rome to inquire about the health of Eugenia Millard, the last person to be cured," Curran, "'Finger of God,'" 55; Pagliarini, "And the Word Was Made Flesh," 216; *Sermons of Father J. P. Clorivière, 1819–1825,* February 10, 1825, Book 9, 20; Stephen Dubuisson, *A Narrative of the Wonderful Cure of Sister Mary Eugenia Millard, a Nun in the Convent of the Visitation, in Georgetown [District of Columbia], on the 10th of February, 1838,* 21, Archives of the Georgetown Visitation Monastery.

54 *Narrative of Two Wonderful Cures,* 8.

55. Ibid., 8, 9.

56. Letter from Ann Mattingly to Stephen Dubuisson, April 16, 1831, Correspondence Extras (210 Extra 64-78), MPA, 64, 7.

57. Ibid.; letter from James Whitfield to Stephen Dubuisson, Baltimore, July 26, 1831, MPA, 64, 7.

58. Ann Mattingly, "Prayers recited by Mrs. Ann Mattingly before and after the cure of her foot, which took place on the 1st of January, 1831 at about 10 1/2 at night in the Convent of the Visitation . . . of Georgetown, D.C.," MPA, 14, 1; "Toast porté au dîner donné par Monsieur Carbery (Washington), à l'occasion du 9me anniversaire de la Guérison Miraculeuse de Madame Mattingly, sa soeur—le 10 Mars 1833," MPA, 14, 1.

59. George Parsons Lathrop and Rose Hawthorne Lathrop, *A Story of Courage, Annals of the Georgetown Convent* (Cambridge, 1895), 289, 307, 308; letter from Stephen Dubuisson to Rev. McCarthy (of Philadelphia), July 2, 1835, MPA, 65, 4 ("living miracle").

Chapter 7. Conclusion

1. England, *Works,* vol. I, 149; personal correspondence, May 3, 2006.

2. The names of the Mattingly and Carbery descendents have been changed to protect their privacy. Valerie MacNess, "Family Bible Yields New Evidence in Famed Mattingly 'Miracle' Cure," *Washington Catholic Sentinel,* February 26, 1965; e-mail communication with Philip M. Hannan, July 15, 2005.

3. *United States Census, 1840,* District of Columbia, Roll 35, 73.

4. *National Intelligencer,* April 23, 1848, says that Annie Elizabeth Mattingly was married to William Butler by Rev. Littleton F. Morgan on April 20, 1848; Rev. French S. Evans married Joseph Mattingly and Hannah Reeves on November 20, 1853, according to the *National Intelligencer* of November 30, 1853. Morgan and Evans were Methodist ministers.

5. Wills of Thomas Carbery and Ann Mattingly were obtained from the Office of the Secretary, Office of Public Records, District of Columbia.

6. The DNA test was done on April 3, 2007, by GeneTree DNA Testing Center; "Martin Doyle, 08/04/1830," Record Group 21, Insolvent Case Papers, National Archives and Records Administration, Washington, DC.

7. On the name Doyle as associated with mixed-race ancestry, see "Melungeon," http://freepages.genealogy.rootsweb.ancestry.com/~genbel/may/melungeon .html (accessed August 21, 2010); on the Wesorts, see William Harlen Gilbert Jr., "The Wesorts of Southern Maryland, an Outcasted Group," *Journal of the Washington Academy of Sciences* 35 (1945), 237–246; Edward T. Price, "A Geographic Analysis of White-Negro-Indian Mixtures in the Eastern United States," *Annals of the Association of American Geographers* 43, 2 (1953), 138–

155; Thomas J. Harte, "Social Origins of the Brandywine Population, *Phylon* (1960–), 24, no. 4 (1963): 369–378.

8. Anne Royall, *Sketches of History, Life, and Manners in the United States, by a Traveller* (New Haven, CT, 1826), 31, 101.

9. Letitia Woods Brown, *The Free Negro in the District of Columbia* (New York: Oxford University Press, 1972), 27, 31.

10. Mary Beth Corrigan, "Making the Most of an Opportunity: Slaves and the Catholic Church in Early Washington," *Washington History*, 12, no. 1 (spring/ summer 2000): 90–101, 96. See also Corrigan's essay "The Ties That Bind: The Pursuit of Community and Freedom among Slaves and Free Blacks in the District of Columbia, 1800–1860," in *Southern City, National Ambition: The Growth of Early Washington, D.C., 1800–1860*, ed. Howard Gillette Jr. (Washington, DC: American Architectural Foundation and George Washington University Center for Washington Area Studies, 1995), and Constance McLaughlin Green, *The Secret City: A History of Race Relations in the Nation's Capital* (Princeton, NJ: Princeton University Press, 1967), esp. chapter 2, "The Emergence of a Self-Reliant Negro Community, 1792–1831."

11. Brown, *The Free Negro*, 25. On another famous Catholic mixed-race family of the same era, the Healys, see James M. O'Toole, *Passing for White: Race, Religion, and the Healy Family, 1820–1920* (Amherst: University of Massachusetts Press, 2002). On Washington City as a community where caste differences among free blacks arose, see Audrey Elisa Kerr, *The Paper Bag Principle: Class, Colorism, and Rumor and the Case of Black Washington, D.C.* (Knoxville: University of Tennessee Press, 2006).

12. Estate of Thomas Carbery, Record Group 21, Records of the District Courts of the United States, Equity Case File 37, *Richie v. Richard Lay, et al.,* and Equity Case File 589, *Prather v. Selden, et al.,* National Archives and Records Administration, Washington, DC.

13. *Joshua A. Ritchie and others v. Richard Lay, ex & Helen McSherry and other heirs of Thomas Carbery,* no. 37 equity, Estate of Thomas Carbery.

14. Estate of Thomas Carbery, *Richie v. Richard Lay, et al.,* and *Prather v. Selden, et al.*

15. "Death of Mr. Mattingly," *Prince George's Enquirer,* January 31, 1908, Upper Marlboro, MD.

16. Albert Garreau, *L'Anneau d'Or: Spirituels de L'Allemagne Romantique* (Paris: La Columbe, 1957), 104.

17. Sebastian, *Fürst Alexander von Hohenlohe-Schillingsfürst,* 91.

18. Pachtler, *Biographische Notizen,* 59, translated from a quotation in Koskull, *Wunderglaube und Medizin,* 12.

19. Heinrich Heine, "Bamberg und Würzburg," http://gutenberg.spiegel.de/index .php?id=12&xid=1142&kapitel=21&cHash=5bc879b5622 (accessed August 21, 2010). See also *Complete Poems of Heinrich Heine: A Modern English Version,* ed. Hal Draper (Boston: Suhrkamp/Insel, 1992), 274. The original German follows:

> In beider Weichbild fließt der Gnaden Quelle,
> Und tausend Wunder täglich dort geschehen.
> Umlagert sieht man dort von Kranken stehen
> Den Fürsten, der da heilet auf der Stelle.
>
> Er spricht: "Steht auf und geht!" und flink und schnelle
> Sieht man die Lahmen selbst von hinnen gehen;
> Er spricht: "Schaut auf und sehet!" und es sehen
> Sogar die Blindgebornen klar und helle.
>
> Ein Jüngling naht, von Wassersucht getrieben,
> Und fleht: "Hilf, Wunderthäter, meinem Leibe!"
> Und segnend spricht der Fürst: "Geh hin und schreibe!"
>
> In Bamberg und in Würzburg macht's Spektakel,
> Die Handlung Göbhardt's rufet laut: "Mirakel!"
> Neun Dramen hat der Jüngling schon geschrieben.

20. Garreau, *L'Anneau d'Or,* 114.

21. Cassiodor Franz Joseph Zenger, *Vertrautes Gespräch über die vom Fürsten Alex. v. Hohenlohe gewirkten Heilungen* (Sulzbach, 1823), 17. The idea that no one is seeking the canonization of Prince Hohenlohe is repeated on page 68. On page 70, Zenger calls for a start to the investigative process of canonization.

22. "Review of Missionary Journal of the Rev. Joseph Wolff, Missionary to the Jews," *Gentleman's Magazine* XCIX, I (London, 1829), 333–334; Rev. S. Baring Gould, "Hohenlohe the Wonder-Working Prince," *Gentleman's Magazine* CCLX (London, 1886), 536–547; Sebastian, *Fürst Alexander von Hohenlohe-Schillingsfürst,* 139.

23. Miller, "A Church in Cultural Captivity," 12.

24. Edward Wakin and Joseph F. Scheuer, *The De-Romanization of the American Catholic Church* (New York: Macmillan, 1966); Jay Dolan, *The American*

Catholic Experience (South Bend, IN: University of Notre Dame Press, 1985); Dolan, *The Immigrant Church: New York's Irish and German Catholics 1815–1865* (South Bend, IN: University of Notre Dame Press, 1992); and Dolan, *Catholic Revivalism: The American Experience, 1830–1900* (South Bend, IN: University of Notre Dame Press, 1979).

25. For information about the Carbery farm, Norway, see "With the Rambler," *Sunday Star,* Washington, DC, April 9, 1916; *National Intelligencer,* March 10, 1855.

26. Lathrop and Lathrop, *A Story of Courage,* 293, 300. Lathrop says that the St. Louis Sisters of the Visitation had written to Catharine Carbery and received this response, dated March 22, 1877. The archivist at this monastery informed me that the letter has been lost.

Index

Note: Page numbers in *italics* refer to illustrations.